DASH Diet Book #2019

The Complete DASH Diet Guide for Beginners with 21-Day Meal Plan to Lose Weight and Reduce Blood Pressure, Prevent Disease and Live Healthy

By Dr. Jennifer Steven

Legal & Disclaimer

The information contained in this book and its contents is not designed to replace or take the place of any form of medical or professional advice; and is not meant to replace the need for independent medical, financial, legal or other professional advice or services, as may be required. The content and information in this book has been provided for educational and entertainment purposes only.

The content and information contained in this book has been compiled from sources deemed reliable, and it is accurate to the best of the Author's knowledge, information and belief. However, the Author cannot guarantee its accuracy and validity and cannot be held liable for any errors and/or omissions. Further, changes are periodically made to this book as and when needed. Where appropriate and/or necessary, you must consult a professional (including but not limited to your doctor, attorney, financial advisor or such other professional advisor) before using any of the suggested remedies, techniques, or information in this book.

Upon using the contents and information contained in this book, you agree to hold harmless the Author from and against any damages, costs, and expenses, including any legal fees potentially resulting from the application of any of the information provided by this book. This disclaimer applies to any loss, damages or injury caused by the use and application, whether directly or indirectly, of any advice or information presented, whether for breach of contract, tort, negligence, personal injury, criminal intent, or under any other cause of action.

Table of Contents

Forward

DASH diet stands for Dietary Approaches to Stop Hypertension. It is a simple diet that is highly appreciated as it promotes healthy living. The diet was designed majorly to lower blood pressure and reduce risks involved in heart related illness, cancer, diabetes, osteoporosis, stroke, and healthy weight loss.

The DASH diet is as a result of medical professionals who worked for years on dietary strategies for sustaining normal blood pressure levels and weight loss. The Dash diet was therefore tested, trusted and approved to reduce blood pressure in both individuals who are healthy and those suffering from hypertension by nutritionists and medical professionals. Since our health is greatly affected by what we eat, the right change in diet can change your life for greatness, and dash diet is the way to go. We help maintain our blood pressure when we eat plenty of vegetables, fruits and lean proteins like chicken and fish while minimizing the intake of red meat, processed sugars, salt and unhelpful fats

The DASH diet does not only help in lowering blood pressure, it also aid in weight loss, prevention of heart related diseases, cancer and diabetes due to high intake of vegetables and fruits. The art of minimizing blood pressure naturally without being hospitalized or under medication is attractive to everyone while we enjoy the dash diet whole meals. It is more fulfilling.

Such a cheap combination of dieting practices definitely end up among the most praise dieting approaches all over and so if you would wish to lose weight while lowering your blood pressure, I will recommend for you the Dash diet. Do so by counting the Calories: and you will love it.

This dash diet cook book is designed to help you in planning for your healthy future. The recipes are clear and easy to follow with simple ingredients that won't give you a hard time. Once you understand and follow them promptly, you will be amazed by the outcome. Have a great time with dash diet!

Chapter 1 DASH Diet 101

What is DASH diet?

DASH stands for Dietary Approach to Stop Hypertension. DASH diet has been clinically proven to reduce blood pressure within 2 weeks in individuals following the diet. It is not only known to help manage the blood pressure but is also designed for weight loss programs, helps to prevent heart diseases, stroke, diabetes and some forms of cancer.

Brief History of the DASH Diet

This diet is originally conceived in 1992 as a way to find the right diet to combat rising cases of morbid hypertension among Americans. Today, after years of exhaustive studies by different health institutions, DASH diet promoted by the United States Government not only for people with hypertension but also as a healthy model diet for every American to prevent lifestyle diseases.

The DASH (Dietary Approaches to Stop Hypertension) diet encourages the consumption of more fruits, vegetables, whole grains and low-fat dairy products. The diet also calls for lean meat, fish, poultry, nuts and beans as different sources of protein and advises reduction of salt, sugar, and fats in general. The amount of salt in a day was 3,200 mg maximum from all sources. Sugar was limited to no more than three teaspoons only. Alcohol consumption is limited to no more than two beverages and caffeinated drinks such as coffee and colas are restricted to a total of three beverages per day.

The studies of individuals basing their diet on DASH model, although not wholly vegetarian, can greatly reduce blood pressure by 6 mm Hg in systolic and 3 mm Hg in diastolic in normal persons. For hypertensive individuals, there is a drop of 11 mm Hg and 6 mm Hg respectively. This is a big cut and large gain to prevent further complications such as heart failure, kidney disease, coronary heart disease and hardening of blood arteries. It was universal to men and women with ages of 48 to 83.

This diet is easy to follow, but beware of so-called healthy foods that actually hide sizeable amounts of salt, white sugar and fats. See the packaging for sodium preservatives, corn syrups and saturated fats. DASH diet maintains ideal body weight that is better than sticking to fads that promises extreme weight loss.

Why the DASH Diet Works

Nutrition experts believe that the DASH Diet is effective at reducing blood pressure for the following reasons:

The diet is rich in important vitamins, minerals and antioxidants

It is a diet that is high in fibre with an abundance of low glycaemic index carbohydrates

This type of diet is effective for people wishing to lose abdominal fat

It includes daily servings of whole grains, a variety of raw and lightly cooked vegetables, fresh fruit, low fat dairy foods, lean meat, chicken, fish, as well as healthy fats from nuts and seeds

5 Benefits of the DASH Diet

The Dietary Approaches to Stop Hypertension, or DASH, is proven to lower blood pressure levels. It was designed for hypertensive people by following a set of eating plan that has low sodium or salt levels and minimal saturated fats and cholesterol. However, it is not intended for people who want to lose weight, although this is also possible by lowering calorie intake and doing some exercises. DASH has five benefits to offer if followed strictly.

- **First**, overall fat, saturated fat, and cholesterol levels are reduced. Heart attack, stroke, and other cardiovascular diseases may be prevented because of this .

- **Second**, the increased intake of fruits, vegetables, and low-fat dairy foods also increases lycopene, beta-carotene, and phytochemicals in the body. Phytochemicals help protect the body from cancers and heart diseases, and they can be found in plants.

- **Third**, fiber intake is increased by including whole grain products in the plan. Fiber aids in the digestion of food and the lessening of cholesterol levels as well.

- **Fourth**, the reduction of sodium in one's diet to no more than 1,500 milligrams a day can be an effective treatment for hypertension. The lesser the salt intake, the lower blood pressure becomes. Thus, the risks of atherosclerosis and congestive heart failure are lessened.

- **Fifth**, sweets and beverages high in sugar are avoided. This helps one to lower calorie intake and maintains sugar balance in the body.

In summary, DASH diet is loaded with minerals like magnesium, potassium, calcium, and protein. It doesn't only lower sodium and cholesterol in the body, but it also provides the needed major body nutrients.

Food to Eat

To treat high blood pressure, the diet should be as varied as possible to provide the body with all the nutrients it needs: fiber, Omega-3, quality protein, etc. Dietary measures should be combined with regular physical activity to strengthen their action.

- Fibers

Fibers are preferred under the dash diet, they reduce cholesterol levels and have a protective effect on the cardiovascular system. At each meal, care should be taken to provide one of the following fiber sources:

- Fruits
- Vegetables
- Whole grains
- legumes
- Omega 3

Omega-3s have positive effects on cardiovascular health. They help to thin the blood and regulate the blood pressure and also have an anti-inflammatory effect of the most interesting. At least once a day, one of the following sources of Omega-3 should be included:

- Nut oil
- Linseed oil
- Colza oil
- Mackerel
- sardines
- Herring
- Salmon
- Nuts
- Flax and chia seeds
- Lean and vegetable proteins

Some sources of animal protein are also sources of saturated fat. Care must be taken to choose foods that combine a high level of protein and good quality fatty acids. As part of the dash diet, the following foods should be included as often as possible for optimal protein intake:

- legumes
- Pisces
- Sea food

- Poultry without skin
- Lean cuts of meat
- Tofu
- Vegetable milks and soy yogurt
- Milk and skim milk
- oleaginous

Other recommended foods:

- antioxidants
- Low energy density foods
- Good hydration

Foods to avoid

It is recommended to adopt a salt-free diet more or less strict in case of hypertension. This diet tends to put the cardiovascular system at rest and to avoid all the foods that could harm it such as alcohol, saturated fats, etc. In addition, it will be necessary to avoid risky behavior: tobacco, sedentary or anarchic diet.

❖ Salt

The dash diet is a low salt diet. It is important, as a first step, to stop adding salt to dishes or cooking.Here is a list of salt-rich foods to avoid as part of the diet for high blood pressure:

- Cubic broths
- Spice mixes
- Mustard
- Cheese (limit to 1 serving per day)
- Classic bread
- Meats
- Smoked food

- Canned vegetables and fish
- Industrial sauces
- Industrial salted biscuits (chips for example)

❖ Alcohol

Alcohol has a harmful effect on the arterial walls. It weakens the walls and, combined with the increase in blood pressure, increases the risk of a cardiovascular event. It is therefore not recommended, as part of the diet for high blood pressure, to limit alcohol consumption to one serving per day for both men and women. Red wine seems to be the least harmful alcohol for the heart.

The diet should be low in saturated fats and total fats. A diet high in saturated fats increases the risk of heart disease and hypertension. Fats are important for the absorption of fat-soluble vitamins and help in building the body's immune system. Use of oils like olive oil, rice bran oil, mustard oil should be promoted in each meal and trans fats which are commonly found in processed and fried food should be avoided.

Trans and saturated fats can also prevent the beneficial action of Omega-3. They are, moreover, involved in the process of formation of atherosclerotic. Combined with high blood pressure, they therefore increase the risk of a cardiovascular event. In the context of the dash diet, we therefore tend to limit the following foods:

- Palm oil
- Hydrogenated margarines
- Industrial products
- Ready meals
- Butter, whole cream
- Cheese
- Meats
- Fatty meat

- Fried and breaded products
- Industrial sauces: mayonnaise, béchamel, etc.
- Pastries, pastries and sweet or savory biscuits
- Fast food, pizza, etc.
- Tobacco

Like alcohol, tobacco weakens the arterial walls. Stopping smoking should therefore be one of the first things to do in case of high blood pressure. Do not hesitate to consult a professional to help you during smoking cessation.

DASH Diet for Weight Loss

High blood pressure can be lowered by the DASH Diet plan and by reduced salt intake (sodium). The DASH eating plan also has other benefits, such as lowering LDL (bad) cholesterol, which, along with lowering blood pressure, can reduce your risk for getting heart disease. Each method alone lowers blood pressure, however, the combination of the eating plan and a decreased sodium intake gives the highest benefit and prevents the development of high blood pressure.

The DASH Diet Plan is:

1- Low in saturated fat, cholesterol, and total fat.

2- Rich in fruits, vegetables, and fat-free or low-fat milk and milk products.

3- Includes whole grain products, fish, poultry, and nuts.

4- Low in lean red meat, sweets, added sugars, and sugar-containing beverages compared to the typical American diet.

5- Rich in potassium, magnesium, calcium, protein and fiber (nutrients that are expected to lower blood pressure).

Daily Nutrient Goals of the DASH Plan (for a 2,100 Calorie Plan):

- Total fat: 27% of Calories:

- Saturated fat: 6% of calories

- Protein: 18% of calories

- Carbohydrate: 55% of calories

- Cholesterol: 150 mg

- Sodium: 2,300 mg. the diet offers 2 levels of daily sodium consumption 2,300 and 1,500 milligrams per day. 2,300 milligrams is the highest level acceptable by the National High Blood Pressure Education Program. 1,500 milligram can lower blood pressure further and more recently is more recommended as adequate intake and one that most people should try to achieve. The lower your salt intake is, the lower your blood pressure. Studies have found that the DASH menus containing 2,300 milligrams of sodium can lower blood pressure and that an even lower level of sodium, 1,500 milligrams, can further reduce blood pressure. Current salt consumption in the United States is 4,200 milligrams per day in adult men and 3,300 milligrams per day in adult women.

- Potassium: 4,700 mg

- Calcium: 1,250 mg

- Magnesium: 500 mg

- Fiber: 30 g

DASH Diet for Diabetes

Over time, many diabetes diet - that is, diets developed with a view to helping people with diabetes better manage their diabetes, have been developed, had their heyday and quietly passed away into sunny retirement. Many though remain strong and just as popular as when they were first introduced. But really, how effective though are these diets.

With the list appearing to grow longer by the year, it often leaves a befuddled public wondering where to begin. So I decided to do review of the most popular diets currently on the market and at the end of that review the DASH diet came through as outstanding performers for helping people manage their diabetes. One may want to ask, what exactly makes up a good Diabetic diet? The following therefore are just some of those elements.

It will be low on carbohydrates or at least provide for a way of either balancing out the carbohydrate through the course of the day or "burning" off the excess, as for example, through exercise.

It should be high in dietary fiber which has been proven to have multiple health benefits like having a low glycemic index and helping to lower the probabilities for diseases like heart disease etc.

Low in salt. Salt can lead to hypertension-that is high blood pressure, so cutting it down is a must

Low in fat. Since fat or foods easily converted to fat like sugars can lead to the individual becoming overweight- a risk factor for diabetes, it is often necessary for such food to have a low-fat content.

A good diabetic diet should strive to meet the recommended daily allowance for potassium. Potassium is important because it can help to reverse the negative effects on the circulatory system that salt has.

The DASH diet evidently has all these characteristics and more. The DASH diet is considered to be the best diet to take for a healthy blood pressure.

However that is not as far as its benefits go. The diet has also been found to be equally efficacious as a diabetes diet. In fact in a review of 35 diets carried out by US News and World report ,it came out joint first with The Biggest Loser diet as the best diabetes diet. It has been shown to display both diabetes prevention and control qualities.

On prevention, it has been shown to help individuals lose weight and also keep it off. Since being overweight is a major risk factor for developing Type 2 diabetes, this quality shows it off as a great diabetes diet option.

In addition, the risk factors associated with metabolic syndrome, a condition which increases the chances of developing diabetes is also reduced by a combination of the DASH diet and calorie restriction. As regards control, the results of a small study published in a 2011 edition of Diabetes Care disclosed that Type 2 diabetics following eight weeks on DASH had reduced their levels of A1C and their fasting blood sugar.

Moreover the diet has been found to be more flexible than most, a fact that would make it easier to follow and adjustable, to enable it comply with a doctors dietary advice to his diabetic patient.

Another advantage offered by this diet is the level of its conformity to dietary guidelines. Light as it may seem, this is actually very important because some diets place a restriction on certain foods, thereby leaving the individual potentially deficient in certain nutrients and minerals.

A breakdown of this conformity shows that where fat is concerned, the diet satisfactorily falls within the 20 to 35 percent of daily Calories:. It also meets the 10 percent maximum threshold allocated to saturated fat by falling well below that. It also meets the recommended amount of proteins and carbohydrates.

Where salt is concerned, it has guideline meal caps for this mineral. Both for the recommended daily maximum of 2,300 mg and if you're African-American, are 51 years or older or have hypertension, diabetes or chronic kidney disease, the 1,500 mg limit.

Other nutrients are adequately taken care of also by this diet. Thus the recommended daily intake of 22 to 34 grams fiber for adults is well provided for by this diet. So too is potassium, a nutrient that is marked for its ability to counter salts blood pressure raising qualities, reduce the risk of developing kidney stones and also decrease bone loss. Impressively so because of the difficulty in normally acquiring the recommended daily intake-4,700 mg or the equivalent of eating 11 bananas a day.

Recommended daily intake of Vitamin D for adults who don't get enough sunlight is penciled down at 15 mg. Though, the diet falls just shy of this, it is suggested that this can be easily made up by say a vitamin D fortified cereal.

Calcium so necessary for strong bones and teeth, blood vessel production and muscle function is also adequately taken care of by the diet.

DASH Diet for Osteoporosis

It becomes apparent that a variety of nutrients affects bone health .Promoting intake of single nutrients is not the best approach in osteoporosis prevention and treatment as nutrients occur together in foods. A typical Western diet--containing inadequate amounts of calcium, vegetables, and fruits and large amounts of salt (NaCl)--harms overall health, including bone.The DASH (Dietary Approaches to Stop Hypertension) dietary plan ,which emphasizes intake of vegetables, fruits, and low-fat diary products and avoids consumption of processed foods, fulfills the need for optimal intake of many bone beneficial nutrients

The DASH diet provides the amount of calcium needed by adults up to 50 years of age, necessitating a calcium supplement to meet the higher needs of those over 50 years. It provides the optimal amount of alkaline potassium eｕuivalents through consumption of fruits and vegetables; these foods also supply magnesium, vitamin C, and other antioxidants, all of which play a role in bone metabolism. Polyphenols, such as those in tea (but in many fruits and vegetables also), have been positively associated with bone health.Moreover, the DASH diet provides a reasonable level of sodium intake without having to endure unpalatable foods. Hence, although the DASH diet is designated to control hypertension, it has complementary, beneficial effects on bone health.

DASH Diet for Heart Disease

Diets to reduce high blood pressure focus on reduced sodium intake and weight loss. The DASH diet to avoid high blood pressure is an eating plan that is low in fat, rich in low fat dairy foods, fruits, vegetables and other plant foods. Following diets to reduce high blood pressure may also reduce the risk of developing heart diseases.

Most experts recommend that following DASH while reducing your sodium intake can effectively lower your blood pressure. There are a number of health supplements that can help, as well. Even strict adherence to a diet to avoid high blood pressure may not be enough alone. Other factors should be addressed as well.

There are many factors which contribute to high blood pressure. Smoking, obesity, chronic stress and genetics are among them. Any of these factors can contribute to an increased risk of heart disease, as well.

Quitting smoking is one of the best things that a person can do for their health. Nicotine increases blood pressure. People who have high blood pressure or a tendency towards high blood pressure should not smoke.

Diets to reduce high blood pressure should address the obesity factor. No more than 30% of a person's total caloric intake should come from fat. In the Standard American Diet, sometimes referred to as SAD, the percentage of dietary fat is much higher. Many foods like ground beef are naturally high in fat. Even in lean or extra lean ground beef most of the calories come from fat. Chicken and turkey breast are better choices for the daily diet. Baked or grilled...not breaded or fried.

Regular physical activity is also important. If you follow a diet to avoid high blood pressure, but you are physically inactive, you may still have high blood pressure. Physical activity improves the function of the heart and the blood vessels. People who are physically active have lower resting heart rates and lower blood pressure. Uncontrolled high blood pressure is one of the major risk factors for the development of heart disease and stroke. Likewise, physical inactivity is related to an increased risk for heart disease.

A diet to avoid high blood pressure will require that you limit or cut out alcohol consumption. Alcohol causes a temporary increase in blood pressure that can become chronic. Alcohol also causes an increase in stress, anxiety and depression.

Chronic stress is one of the major risk factors for developing both high blood pressure and heart disease. Stress causes an increase in blood pressure. It is important to learn how to relieve stress on a daily basis. Regular exercise, yoga, meditation and certain dietary supplements can help.

In order to reduce sodium intake, most diets to reduce high blood pressure limit quantities of processed foods. You may not realize how much salt is in processed cheese, peanut butter, salad dressing and other processed foods. Many carbonated beverages are also high in sodium content. Water on the other hand, contains no salt, and is a natural diuretic.

Fluid retention is one of the health problems associated with high blood pressure. Prescription medications for high blood pressure are diuretics, but there are natural diuretics, including most fruits and vegetables. This is one reason that a diet to reduce high blood pressure is rich in fruits and vegetables. In particular, watermelon, citrus fruits, lettuce, celery and low-fat cottage cheese have a natural diuretic effect and can help you lose water weight. Salt and alcohol cause the body to retain more fluid. After a night of eating chips and drinking beer, you will typically find that you weigh about three more pounds than you did the day before.

Although the Dietary Approaches to Stop Hypertension (DASH) diet was developed to help prevent and treat hypertension, the foods that make up the diet protect and sustain your health in many ways:

DASH is low in red meat. In fact, you could cut out red meat altogether, if you prefer. This is important for cancer prevention because a high intake of red meat and processed meats is linked to cancers of the colon, rectum, esophagus, stomach, prostate, lung, and kidney.

DASH is rich in fruits and vegetables. People who eat little in the way of fruits and vegetables double their risk of cancers of the lung, mouth, throat, esophagus, breast, pancreas, stomach, colon, rectum, cervix, and bladder compared with those whose intake of fruits and vegetables tracks closely with DASH.

DASH emphasizes low-fat dairy products. The impact of dairy foods on cancer risk is less clear than it is for other foods. There is evidence that eating a lot of high-fat dairy foods compared to choosing low-fat or non-fat dairy products may raise breast cancer risk. Other studies have found a lower risk for colon cancer with dairy foods.Until the medical community knows more, men concerned about prostate cancer risk should probably limit low-fat dairy to 2 servings or fewer on average per day.

NOTE :When it comes to prostate cancer, the data gets rather murky. A high intake of whole-fat dairy products (more than 2-1/2 servings per day) is strongly correlated with prostate cancer, whereas the connection appears to be weaker with low-fat dairy. One study of men with prostate cancer found that those who ate the least amount of yogurt were more apt to have more aggressive cancers.

DASH has plenty of whole grains. Whole grains are great for the digestive tract, with good evidence of protection against colorectal, pancreatic, and stomach cancer. Although the connection isn't clear, some studies suggest that whole grains may help prevent breast cancer.

DASH includes moderate amounts of nuts, seeds, and beans. Beans may make you feel a little gassy, but they're nutrient powerhouses and will keep your colon happy, cutting your risk for cancers of the colon, pancreas, and breast.

And although you may think of nuts and seeds as high-fat foods, they mainly supply healthy monounsaturated and polyunsaturated fats (including omega-3) and little in the way of the more harmful saturated fats.

Studies of nut consumption have pointed to a more than 10 percent drop in cancer incidence, including colon, breast, and prostate, in people who enjoy nuts regularly. Of course, you don't want to go nuts with nuts. Those Calories: aren't freebies, so it's best to stick to the DASH guidelines.

DASH limits fats and oils. A diet high in saturated fats, lard, bacon grease, and butter is clearly linked to cancer risk, including cancers of the breast, colon, and pancreas.

Less is known about the saturated fats from tropical oils such as coconut oil and palm oil, so until scientists know more, you can't assume that tropical oils are safer. Trans fats, including those from solid margarine and vegetable shortening, appear to increase your risk for lymphoma.

DASH keeps sweets to a minimum. Although sugar itself doesn't appear to cause cancer, sugary foods tend to be low in healthy nutrients. By choosing a sugary snack rather than a piece of fruit or a handful of nuts, you simultaneously deprive yourself of something that's really good for you and fill your body with empty Calories:.

Chapter 3 Fllow the DASH Meal Plan

Who Should follow a DASH Meal plan?

In fact, a DASH eating plan can be a part of any healthy eating plan. Not only, will it help lower blood pressure but it will offer additional heart health benefits including lowering LDL cholesterol and inflammation.

How to Fllow the DASH Diet

Reducing Salts And Sodium

With the approach of ingesting more fruits and vegetables in DASH eating plan, it has made it easier to consume less salt and sodium conseuently owing to its lower content of sodium. In addition, fruits and vegetables are potassium-rich diet which plays a role in reducing high blood pressure. Others common dietary sources are milk products and fish.

There are some tips to reduce the sodium:

- Restrict salt-rich containing foods. It is preferably to take no or low-salt-added foods.
- Increased intake of vegetables.
- No salt-added rice, noodles or any other mixed dishes
- Removing excess salt from preserved food such as tuna or beans which are being preserved in a can form.

Friendly cooking methods

✓ Use healthy cooking techniques

Unhealthy cooking habits can sabotage your other efforts to stick to the DASH diet. Use these tips to help reduce sodium and fat:

- **Spice it up.** Enhance flavor without adding salt or fat by using herbs, spices, flavored vinegars, onions, peppers, ginger, lemon, garlic or garlic powder, or sodium-free bouillon.
- **Rinse it off.** Rinse canned foods, such as beans and vegetables, before using to wash away some excess salt.
- **Beware of broth.** You can cook mushrooms, onions or other vegetables in a little low-sodium broth in a nonstick pan. But because even low-sodium broth can have lots of sodium, a little healthy oil may be a better option.
- **Make lower fat substitutions.** Replace full-fat dairy with reduced-fat or fat-free versions.
- **Cut back on meat.** Prepare stews and casseroles with only two-thirds of the meat the recipe calls for, and add extra vegetables, brown rice, tofu, bulgur or whole-wheat pasta.
- If you tend to cook or bake in ways that call for lots of fat and salt, don't be afraid to modify your recipes. Experiment with spices and substitutions. Branch out and try recipes you wouldn't normally try. You may be pleasantly surprised by what you create!

Choose the right cookware

Your cookware and kitchen gadgets can make it easier to follow the DASH diet. Helpful items include:

- Nonstick cookware. Nonstick cookware reduces the need to use oil or butter when sauteing meat or vegetables.
- Vegetable steamer. A vegetable steamer that fits in the bottom of a pan makes it easy to prepare vegetables without butter or oil.
- Spice mill or garlic press. These items make it easy to add flavor to your food and reduce your dependence on the shaker of salt.

Excise More

You can lose weight while following the DASH diet plan at lower calorie levels with increasing your physical activity. The best way to lose weight is by doing so gradually, getting more physical activity, and eating a balanced diet that is lower in Calories: and fat.

Physical activity can be done at one time for 30 minutes , or at 3 times 10 minutes each for a total of 30 minutes. To avoid weight gain, try to total about 60 minutes per day.

How to Do in Our Daily Life

This diet, coined as the 'Healthiest Diet', is designed to provide real-life solutions to high-blood pressure by suggesting a diet that merely regulates the intake of nutrients and not alter the common diet we're all used to. Dietary Approaches to Stop Hypertension or dash focuses on controlling the intake of sodium and fats to maintain the normal blood pressure of an individual. Dash is geared towards preparing a diet that makes satisfying meals, thus, preventing people from eating in-between meals, causing loss of control over food intake. Because it keeps people from hunger in-between meals, it ideally becomes more satisfying and less controlling.

The Dash diet teaches individuals to complete the whole dash diet program by starting with stocking up the kitchen with dash-friendly food, preparing dash-friendly recipes, and performing Dash-friendly exercises. Meal plans suggested by Dash usually contain ingredients high in fibre, calcium, magnesium and potassium. Dash diets go low on sodium and sugar and emphasize the need to eat green leafy vegetables and fruits.

Avocado dip, for instance, is one of the most famous Dash diets there is today, because of its very convenient and affordable preparation. Avocado, a very rich source of monosaturated fat and lutein, (antioxidants that help protect vision), is among the many fruits that are highly-recommended for Dash diet.

In this recipe, avocado has to be mashed and pitted, mixed with fat-free sour cream, onion and hot sauce. This dip shall be eaten with tortilla chips or sliced vegetables. From this dish, a person can get a total of 65 calories, 2 grams protein, 5 grams total fat, 4 grams carbohydrate, 172 milligrams potassium and 31 milligrams calcium. From this we can infer that a person is fed a considerable amount of necessary nutrients, essential for maintaining a well-balanced diet that's good for the heart.

In just 14 days, a Dash diet follower will experience normal blood pressure, with fewer tendencies to eat in-between meals, the major culprit of weight gain. The Dash diet program also teaches individuals to determine the right amount of food intake, the necessary exercise to perform according to age and activity level. Dash educates and motivates --- one of the very important reasons why people find it easy to stick to the diet. Also, the diet does not re□uire us to give up anything significant in our usual diet, instead, it helps us create a process of adjusting to little changes so we can successfully help ourselves.

Tips on Following DASH When Eating Out

When eating out at restaurants, these tips can help you order the best options for your high blood pressure:

Try foods like:

- Grilled, roasted, broiled menu items
- Fresh fruits and vegetables as sides
- Spices and fresh herbs, which do not contain sodium (basil, garlic, curry powder, etc.)
- Fresh vegetables for pizza and burger toppings
- Vegetarian dishes
- Fresh fruits or sorbets for dessert
- Limit or avoid foods that tend to be higher in sodium:

- Meats that are fried, smoked, cured, or processed
- Condiments like mustard, ketchup, pickles, and soy sauce
- Most soups
- Additives like MSG
- Dishes like rice pilaf, casserole-style dishes, charcuterie plates (cheese, cured meats, olives)

Don't be afraid to:

- Ask for the nutrition information (specifically sodium) for any foods you are unsure about.
- Ask that less or no salt be added to your dish.
- Ask for dressings and sauces on the side to help control the amount of sodium you'll be ingesting.
- Most importantly… taste your food before you season it!
- Don't let high blood pressure stop you from enjoying dining out with friends and family. With these easy changes, you can manage your health deliciously! Work with your doctor and/or a registered dietitian to stay on track with a diet to lower blood pressure.

1. Are Eggs on the DASH Diet?

Yes . Eggs are also included in the dash diet

2. Can I Follow DASH if I am a Vegetarian?

Yes, DASH can be adapted to a vegetarian eating pattern. In fact, the DASH diet was originally created based on a vegetarian diet because we know that vegetarians tend to have lower blood pressures. The diet used in the research that demonstrated the efficacy of DASH did include animal protein foods, such as meat, poultry, fish, and dairy foods. But we are confident that similar health benefits can be obtained using vegetable sources of protein and dairy foods. Remember that DASH includes lots of fruits and vegetables, low fat dairy foods, and limited added fats and oils. These recommendations are the same for vegetarians and fish, meat, and poultry eaters. In order to meet your DASH food goals for meats we suggest you substitute with the nuts, seeds and legumes category. Simply add your recommended servings of meat to your recommended servings of legumes and aim for that goal every day.

3. I'm taking medications. Could this diet affect how they work?

Certain medications, like blood thinners or medications for diabetes, can have an interaction with the foods you eat. If you're on medications, discuss with your doctor whether dramatically changing your diet will affect how your medications work before starting the diet.

Chapter 4 Breakfast Recipes

Very Berry Muesli

Prep time: 10 mins | Servings: 2

Ingredients:

- 1 c. Oats
- 1 c. Fruit flavored Yogurt
- ½ c. Milk
- 1/8 tsp. Salt
- ½ c dried Raisins
- ½ c. chopped Apple
- ½ c. frozen Blueberries
- ¼ c. chopped Walnuts

Directions:

1. Combine your yogurt, salt, and oats together in a medium bowl, mix well, and then cover the mixture tightly.
2. Allow to rest in the refrigerator for at least 6 hours. Add your raisins, and apples the gently fold.
3. Top with walnuts and serve. Enjoy!

Nutritional Information:

Calories: 195 Protein 6g, Carbs 31g, Fat 4g.

Veggie Quiche Muffins

Prep time: 10 mins | Servings: 12

Ingredients:

- ¾ c. shredded Cheddar
- 1 c. chopped Green Onion
- 1 c. chopped Broccoli
- 1 c. diced Tomatoes
- 2 c. Milk
- 4 Eggs
- 1 c. Pancake mix
- 1 tsp. Oregano
- ½ tsp. Salt
- ½ tsp. Pepper

Directions:

1. Preheat your oven to 375 degrees F, and lightly grease a 12-cup muffin tin with oil. Sprinkle your tomatoes, broccoli, onions, and cheddar into your muffin cups.
2. Combine your remaining ingredients in a medium, whisk to combine then pour evenly on top of your veggies.
3. Set to bake in your preheated oven for about 40 minutes or until golden brown. Allow to cool slightly (about 5 minutes) then serve. Enjoy!

Nutritional Information:

Calories: 58.5 Protein 5.1 g, Carbs 2.9 g, Fat 3.2 g.

Turkey Sausage and Mushroom Strata

Prep time: 10 mins | Servings: 12

Ingredients:

- 8 oz. cubed Ciabatta bread
- 12 oz. chopped Turkey sausage
- 2 c. Milk
- 4 oz. shredded Cheddar
- 3 large Eggs
- 12 oz. Egg substitute
- ½ c. chopped Green onion
- 1 c. diced Mushroom
- ½ tsp. Paprika
- ½ tsp. Pepper
- 2 tbsps. grated Parmesan cheese

Directions:

1. Set oven to preheat to 400 degrees F.
2. Lay your bread cubes flat on a baking tray and set it to toast for about 8 min. Meanwhile, add a skillet over medium heat with sausage, and allow to cook, while stirring, until fully brown and crumbled.
3. In a large bowl add salt, pepper, paprika, parmesan cheese, egg substitute, eggs, cheddar cheese, and milk, then whisk to combine.
4. Add in your remaining ingredients and toss well to incorporate.
5. Transfer mixture to a large baking dish (preferably a 9x13-inch) then tightly cover and allow to rest in the refrigerator overnight.
6. Set your oven to preheat to 350 degrees, remove the cover from your casserole and set to bake until golden brown and cooked through.
7. Slice and serve.

Nutritional Information:

Calories: 288.2 Protein 24.3g, Carbs 18.2g, Fat. 12.4g.

Bacon bits

Prep time: 15 mins | Servings: 4

Ingredients:

- 1 c. Millet
- 5 c. Water
- 1 c. diced Sweet potato
- 1 tsp. ground Cinnamon
- 2 tbsps. Brown sugar
- 1 medium diced Apple
- ¼ c. Honey

Directions:

1. In a deep pot, add your sugar, sweet potato, cinnamon, water, and millet then stir to combine.
2. Allow to come to a boil over high heat then reduce to a simmer on low.
3. Cook like this for about an hour, on until your water is fully absorbed and millet is cooked.
4. Stir in your remaining ingredients, and serve.

Nutritional Information:

Calories: 136 Protein 3.1g, Carbs 28.5g, Fat 1.0g.

Summer Breakfast Quinoa Bowls

Prep time: 5 mins | Servings: 2

Ingredients:

- 1 sliced Peach
- 1/3 c. Quinoa
- 1 c. Low fat milk
- ½ tsp. Vanilla extract
- 2 tsps. Brown sugar
- 12 Raspberries
- 14 Blueberries
- 2 tsps. Honey

Directions:

1. Add brown sugar, 2/3 cup milk, and quinoa to a saucepan, and stir to combine.
2. Over medium heat, bring to a boil then cover and reduce heat to a low simmer.
3. Continue to cook for about 20 minutes (you should be able to fluff quinoa with a fork).
4. Grease and preheat your grill to medium and grill your peach slices for about a minute per side then set aside.
5. Reheat your remaining milk in the microwave and set aside.
6. Split your cooked quinoa evenly between 2 serving bowls and top evenly with your remaining ingredients. Enjoy!

Nutritional Information:

Calories: 180 Protein 4.5 g, Carbs 36g, Fat 4g.

Strawberry Breakfast Sandwich

Prep time: 5 mins | Servings: 4

Ingredients:

- 8 oz. Cream cheese
- 1 tbsp. Honey
- 1 tbsp. grated Lemon zest
- 4 sliced English muffins
- 2 c. sliced Strawberries

Directions:

1. Add your honey, lemon zest, and cheese to a food processor, and process until fully incorporated.
2. Use your cheese mixture to spread on your English muffins as you would butter.
3. Top with strawberries. Enjoy!

Nutritional Information:

Calories: 180 Protein 2g, Carbs 9g, Fat 16g.

Steel Cut Oat Blueberry Pancakes

Prep time: 5 mins | Servings: 4

Ingredients:

- 1½ c. Water
- ½ c. steel cut Oats
- 1/8 tsp. Salt
- 1 c. whole wheat Flour
- ½ tsp. Baking powder
- ½ tsp. Baking soda
- 1 Egg
- 1 c. Milk
- ½ c. Greek yogurt
- 1 c. frozen Blueberries
- ¾ c. Agave Nectar

Directions:

1. Combine your oats, salt, and water together in a medium saucepan, stir, and allow to come to a boil over high heat.
2. Lower heat, and allow to simmer for about 10 min, or until oats get tender. Set aside.
3. Combine all your remaining ingredients, except agave nectar, in a medium bowl then fold in oats.
4. Preheat your griddle, and lightly grease.
5. Cook ¼ cup of batter at a time for about 3 minutes per side.
6. Garnish with agave.

Nutritional Information:

Calories: 257 Protein 14g, Carbs 46g, Fat 7g.

Spinach, Mushroom, and Feta Cheese Scramble

Prep time: 3 mins | Servings: 1

Ingredients:

- Olive oil cooking spray
- ½ c. sliced Mushroom
- 1 c. chopped Spinach
- 3 Eggs
- 2 tbsps. Feta cheese
- Pepper

Directions:

1. Set a lightly greased, medium skillet over medium heat.
2. Add spinach, and mushrooms, and cook until spinach wilts.
3. Combine egg whites, cheese, pepper, and whole egg together in a medium bowl then whisk to combine.
4. Pour into your skillet and cook, while stirring, until set (about 4 minutes).
5. Serve.

Nutritional Information:

Calories: 236.5 Protein 22.2g, Carbs 12.9g, Fat 11.4g.

Refrigerator Overnight Oatmeal

Prep time: 5 mins | Servings: 2

Ingredients:

- 1c. Oats
- 1 c. Non-fat yogurt
- ½ c. Milk
- 1 c. frozen Blueberries
- 1 tbsp. Chia seeds

Directions:

1. Add all your ingredients to a medium mixing bowl, and stir.
2. Split evenly among 2 airtight containers, seal, and refrigerate overnight.
3. Serve.

Nutritional Information:

Calories: 244 Protein 16g, Carbs 37g, Fat 5g.

Red Velvet Pancakes with Cream Cheese Topping

Prep time: 15 mins | Servings: 2

Ingredients:

Cream Cheese Topping:

- 2 oz. Cream cheese
- 3 tbsps. Yogurt
- 3 tbsps. Honey
- 1 tbsp. Milk

Pancakes:

- ½ c. whole wheat Flour
- ½ c. all-purpose Flour
- 2¼tsps. Baking powder
- ½ tsp. unsweetened Cocoa powder
- ¼ tsp. Salt
- ¼ c. Sugar
- 1 large Egg
- 1 c. + 2 tbsps. Milk
- 1 tsp. Vanilla
- 1 tsp. Red paste food coloring

Directions:

1. Combine all your topping ingredients in a medium bowl, and set aside.
2. Add all your pancake ingredients together in a large bowl and fold until combined.
3. Set a greased skillet over medium heat to get hot.
4. Add ¼ cup of pancake batter onto the hot skillet and cook until bubbles begin to form on the top.
5. Flip and cook until set. Repeat until your batter is done.
6. Add your toppings and serve.

Nutritional Information:

Calories: 231 Protein 7g, Carbs 43g, Fat 4g.

Perfect Granola

Prep time: 10 mins | Servings: 10

Ingredients:

- ¼ c. Canola oil
- 4 tbsps. Honey
- 1½ tsps. Vanilla
- 6 c. Old fashioned rolled oats
- 1 c. Almond
- ½ c. shredded coconut
- 2 c. Bran flakes
- ¾ c. chopped Walnuts
- 1 c. Raisins
- Cooking spray

Directions:

1. Prepare oven to preheat at 325 degrees F.
2. In a saucepan cook oil and vanilla gently over low flame, occasionally stirring for roughly 5 mins.
3. Place all (except raisins) ingredients remaining, in a large bowl and combine.
4. Stir in honey and oil mixture slowly and ensure that all grains are properly coated.
5. Cover a baking tray with parchment paper or use cooking spray to spray it lightly. Spread cereal evenly in the tray and bake for 25 mins occasionally stirring to keep mixture from burning), or until very lightly browned, or the grains crisp.
6. When finished, remove cereal and put to cool.
7. Add the cup of raisins and mix well so that raisins are thoroughly spread through the grain mixture.

Nutritional Information:

Calories: 458 Protein 12.1g, Carbs 62g, Fat 21g.

Peanut Butter & Banana Breakfast Smoothie

Prep time: 2 mins | Servings: 1

Ingredients:

- 1 c. Non-fat milk
- 1 tbsp. Peanut butter
- 1 Banana
- ½ tsp. Vanilla

Directions:

1. Place, non-fat milk, peanut butter and banana in a blender.
2. Blend until smooth.

Nutritional Information:

Calories: 295 Protein 133g, Carbs 42g, Fat 8.4g.

Overnight Oatmeal

Prep time: 6 mins | Servings: 8

Ingredients:

- 4 c. Fat-free milk
- 4 c. Water
- 2 c. Steel-cut oats
- 1/3 c. Cup raisins
- 1/3 c. Dried cherries
- 1/3 c. Dried apricots
- 1 tsp. Molasses
- 1 tsp. Cinnamon
- ½ tsp. Nutmeg

Directions:

1. Combine all ingredients in a slow cooker.
2. Turn on low heat. Seal lid, cook for 8 to 9 hours overnight.
3. Ladle into bowls. Serve.

Nutritional Information:

Calories: 114 Protein 6g, Carbs 20g, Fat 1g, sodium 44.0.

No Bake Breakfast Granola Bars

Prep time: 3 mins | Servings: 18

Ingredients:

- 2 c. Old fashioned oatmeal
- ½ c. Raisins
- ½ c. Brown sugar
- 2½ c. Corn rice cereal
- ½ c. Syrup
- ½ c. Peanut butter
- ½ tsp. Vanilla

Directions:

1. In a suitable size mixing bowl, mix together using a wooden spoon, rice cereal, oatmeal, and raisins.
2. In a saucepan, combine corn syrup and brown sugar.
3. On medium-high flame constantly stir mixture and bring to a boil.
4. On boiling, take away from heat.
5. In a saucepan, stir vanilla and peanut into the sugar mixture. Stir until very smooth.
6. Spoon peanut butter mixture on the cereal and raisins into the mixing bowl and combine. Shape mixture into a 9 x 13 baking tin.
7. Allow to cool properly then cut into bars (18 pcs).

Nutritional Information:

Calories: 152 Protein 4g, Carbs 26g, Fat 4.3g.

Mushroom Shallot Frittata

Prep time: 3 mins | Servings: 4

Ingredients:

- 1 tsp. Butter
- 4 chopped Shallots
- ½ lb. chopped Mushrooms
- 2 tsps. Chopped parsley
- 1 tsp. Dried thyme
- Black pepper
- 3 medium Eggs
- 5 large Egg whites
- 1 tbsp. Milk
- ¼ c. grated parmesan cheese

Directions:

1. Heat oven to 350 degrees.
2. In a suitable size oven-proof skillet, heat butter over medium flame.
3. Add shallots and sauté for about 5 mins. or until golden brown.
4. Add to pot, thyme, parsley, chopped mushroom and black pepper to taste.
5. Whisk milk, egg whites, parmesan and eggs into a bowl.
6. Pour mixture into the skillet ensuring the mushroom is totally covered.
7. Transfer the skillet to the oven as soon as the edges begin to set.
8. Bake until frittata is cooked (15-20 mins).
9. Should be served warm, cut into equal wedges (4 pcs).

Nutritional Information:

Calories: 346 Protein 19.1g, Carbs 48.3g, Fat 12g.

Jack-o-Lantern Pancakes

Prep time: 6 mins | Servings: 8

Ingredients:

- 1 Egg
- ½ c. Canned pumpkin
- 1¾c. Low-fat milk
- 2 tbsps. Vegetable oil
- 2 c. Flour
- 2 tbsps. Brown sugar
- 1 tbsp. Baking powder
- 1 tsp. Pumpkin pie spice
- 1 tsp. Salt

Directions:

1. In a mixing bowl, mix milk, pumpkin, eggs, and oil.
2. Add dry ingredients to egg mixture. Stir gently.
3. Coat griddle lightly with cooking spray and heat on medium.
4. When the griddle is hot, spoon (using a dessert spoon) batter onto griddle.
5. When bubbles start bursting, flip pancakes over and cook until it's a nice golden-brown color.

Nutritional Information:

Calories: 313 Protein 15g, Carbs 28g, Fat 16g.

Morning Quinoa

Prep time: 10 mins | Servings: 4

Ingredients:

- 2 c. Non-fat milk
- 1 c. Quinoa
- ¼ c. Brown sugar
- ½ tsp. Cinnamon
- ¼ c. sliced Slivered almonds
- ¼ c. Dried currants

Directions:

1. Wash the quinoa properly. In a saucepan, bring milk to a boil.
2. Bring the milk to a boil in a medium saucepan.
3. Add quinoa and continue boiling. Cover pot and bring flame to low and simmer until most of the liquid is dissolved (about 15 mins).
4. Turn off heat and use a fork to fluff. Add other ingredients and mix well.
5. Cover and put aside for 15 mins.

Nutritional Information:

Calories: 287 Protein 10.2g, Carbs 52g, Fat 5g.

Fruit-n-Grain Breakfast Salad

Prep time: 2 mins | Servings: 6

Ingredients:

- 3 c. Water
- ¼ tsp. Salt
- ¾ c. Brown rice
- ¾ c. Bulgur
- 1 diced Green apple
- 1 diced Red apple
- 1 Orange
- 1 c. Raisins
- 8 oz. Vanilla yogurt

Directions:

1. Over high flame, boil water in a large pot.
2. Add the bulgur and the rice, lower flame. Close lid and allow cooking time of 10 mins.
3. After cooking, remove from heat, cover for 2 mins; set aside.
4. On a baking sheet, lay hot grains to cool (will give you a fluffier look). Can be prepared overnight and refrigerate.
5. Prepare fruit; core and dice your apples, just before serving. Peel and section your orange.
6. Remove chilled grains from refrigerator; transfer to a medium size mixing bowl, add cut fruit.
7. Mix in yogurt into grains until well coated.

Nutritional Information:

Calories: 116 Protein 3g, Carbs 24.5g, Fat 1g.

Fruit Pizza

Prep time: 3 mins | Servings: 2

Ingredients:

- 1 English muffin
- 2 tbsps. Fat-free cream cheese
- 2 tbsps. sliced strawberries
- 2 tbsps. blueberries
- 2 tbsps. crushed pineapple

Directions:

1. Cut English muffin in half and toast halves until slightly browned.
2. Coat both halves with cream cheese.
3. Arrange fruits atop cream cheese on muffin halves.
4. Serve soon after prepared.
5. Any leftovers refrigerate within 2 hours.

Nutritional Information:

Calories: 119 Protein 6g, Carbs 23g, Fat 1g.

Flax Banana Yogurt Muffins

Prep time: 10 mins | Servings: 12

Ingredients:

- 1 c. Whole wheat flour
- 1 c. Old-fashioned rolled oats
- 1 tsp. Baking soda
- 2 tbsps. Ground flaxseed
- 3 large ripe bananas
- ½ c. Greek yogurt
- ¼ c. Unsweetened applesauce
- ¼ c. Brown sugar
- 2 tsps. Vanilla extract

Directions:

1. Set oven at 355 degrees F and preheat.
2. Prepare muffin tin (can use cooking spray or cupcake liners.
3. Combine dry ingredients in a mixing bowl.
4. In a separate bowl, mix yogurt, banana, sugar, vanilla, and applesauce.
5. Combine both mixtures and mix. Do not over mix. Batter should not be smooth but lumpy.
6. Bake for 20 mins. or when inserted toothpick comes out clean.

Nutritional Information:

Calories: 136 Protein 4g, Carbs 30g, Fat 2g.

Chapter 5 Lunch Recipes

Veggie Quesadillas with Cilantro Yogurt Dip

Prep time: 20 mins | Servings: 3

Ingredients:

- 1 c. Black Beans
- 2 tbsps. chopped Cilantro
- ½ chopped Bell pepper
- ½ c. Corn kernels
- 1 c. shredded Cheese
- 6 Corn tortillas
- 1 shredded Carrot
- ½ minced Jalapeno pepper

Directions:

1. Set your skillet to preheat on low heat.
2. Lay 3 tortillas on a flat surface. Top evenly with peppers, carrots, cilantro, beans, corn, and cheese over the tortillas (covering each with another tortilla, maximum.
3. Add your quesadilla to your preheated skillet, and cook until the cheese melts, and tortilla becomes a nice golden brown (about 2 min).
4. Flip to quesadilla, and cook for about a minute (or until golden).
5. Mix well. Slice each quesadilla into 4 even wedges, and serve with your dip. Enjoy!

Nutritional Information:

Calories: 344 Protein 27g, Carbs 46g, Fat 8g.

Sweet Roasted Beet & Arugula Tortilla Pizza

Prep time: 10 mins | Servings: 6

Ingredients:

- 2 chopped Beets
- 6 Corn Tortillas
- 1 c. Arugula
- ½ c. Goat cheese
- 1 c. Blackberries
- 2 tbsps. Honey
- 2 tbsps. Balsamic vinegar

Directions:

1. Set your oven to preheat to 350 F.
2. Lay your tortillas on a flat surface. Top with beets, berries, and goat cheese.
3. Combine your balsamic vinegar, and honey together in a small bowl, and whisk to combine.
4. Drizzle the mixture over your pizza, and to bake for about 10 minutes, or until your cheese has melted slightly, and your tortilla crisp.
5. Garnish with arugula, and serve.

Nutritional Information:

Calories: 286 Protein 15g, Carbs 42g, Fat 40g.

Sunshine Wrap

Prep time: 20 mins | Servings: 4

Ingredients:

- 8 oz. Grilled chicken breast
- ½ c. diced Celery
- 2/3 c. Mandarin oranges
- ¼ c. minced Onion
- 2 tbsps. Mayonnaise
- 1 tp. Soy sauce
- ¼ tsp. Garlic powder
- ¼ tsp. Black pepper
- 1 large whole wheat Tortilla
- 4 Lettuce leaves

Directions:

1. Combine all your ingredients, except tortilla, and lettuce in a large bowl and toss to evenly coat.
2. Lay your tortillas down on a flat surface and cut into quarters.
3. Top each quarter with a lettuce leaf, and spoon your chicken mixture into the middle of each.
4. Roll each tortilla into a cone and seal by slightly wetting the edge with water. Enjoy!

Nutritional Information:

Calories: 280.8 Protein19g, Carbs 3g, Fat 21.1g.

Southwestern Black Bean Cakes with Guacamole

Prep time: 15 mins | Servings: 4

Ingredients:

- 1 c. Whole wheat bread crumbs
- 3 tbsps. chopped Cilantro
- 2 garlic cloves
- 15 oz. Black beans
- 7 oz. Chipotle peppers in Adobo sauce
- 1 tsp. ground Cumin
- 1 large Egg
- ½ medium diced Avocado
- 1 tbsp. Lime juice
- 1 small tomato

Directions:

1. Drain beans then add all your ingredients, except avocado, lime juice, and eggs, to a food processor and run until the mixture begin to pull away from the sides of processor.
2. Transfer to a large bowl, and add in egg then mix well.
3. Form into 4 even patties, and cook on a preheated, greased grill over medium heat for about 10 minutes, flipping halfway through.
4. Add your avocado, and lime juice in a small bowl, then stir and mash together using a fork.
5. Season to taste then serve with bean cakes.

Nutritional Information:

Calories: 178 Protein 11g, Carbs 25g, Fat 7g.

Southwest Style Rice Bowl

Prep time: 5 mins | Servings: 2

Ingredients:

- 1 tbsp. Vegetable oil
- 1 c. Chopped vegetables
- 1 c. chopped Chicken breast
- 1 c. Brown rice
- 4 tbsps. Salsa
- 2tbsps. shredded Cheddar cheese
- 2 tbsps. Sour cream

Directions:

1. Set a skillet with oil to heat up over medium heat.
2. Add chopped vegetables and allow to cook, while stirring, until vegetables become fork tender.
3. Add chicken, and brown rice and continue to cook, while stirring, until fully heated through.
4. Split between 2 serving bowls, and garnish with your remaining ingredients. Serve, and enjoy!

Nutritional Information:

Calories: 168 Protein 5.5g, Carbs 18g, Fat 8.2g.

Pear, Turkey and Cheese Sandwich

Prep time: 3 mins | Servings: 2

Ingredients:

- 2 slices of Bread
- 2 tsps. Dijon Mustard
- 2 slices smoked Turkey
- 1 sliced Pear
- ¼ c. shredded Mozzarella cheese
- 1/8 tsp. ground Pepper

Directions:

1. Use your mustard to spread on both slices of bread, then top each side with turkey and set one side aside.
2. Top your remaining half with pear slices, and season with pepper.
3. Close your sandwich, and set to broil for about 3 minutes, or until your cheese has been melted, and turkey warmed.
4. Enjoy!

Nutritional Information:

Calories: 337.3 Protein 16.5g, Carbs 55.8g, Fat 11.6g

Salmon Salad Pita

Prep time: 5 mins | Servings: 3

Ingredients:

- ¾ c. Salmon
- 3 tbsps. Yoghurt
- 1 tbsp. Lemon juice
- 2 tbsps. minced Bell pepper
- 1 tbsp. minced Red Onion
- 1 tsp. chopped Capers
- 1 tsp. dried Dill
- 3 Lettuce
- Black pepper
- 3 whole wheat Pita bread

Directions:

1. In a bowl, create your salmon salad by combining your first 8 ingredients, then stir.
2. Create salmon pita by spooning your salmon salad evenly onto your letter leaf then placing it inside your pitas.
3. Enjoy!

Nutritional Information:

Calories: 239 Protein 25g, Carbs 19g, Fat 7g.

Pesto & Mozzarella Stuffed Portobello Mushroom Caps

Prep time: 15 mins | Servings: 2

Ingredients:

- 2 Portobello caps Mushrooms
- 1 small diced tomato
- 2 tbsps. Pesto
- ¼ c. shredded Mozzarella cheese

Directions:

1. Spoon your pesto into evenly into your mushroom caps, then to with your remaining ingredients.
2. Set to bake at 400 degrees F for about 15 minutes.
3. Enjoy!

Nutritional Information:

Calories: 112 Protein 10.5g, Carbs 7.5g, Fat 5.4g.

Fresh Shrimp Spring Rolls

Prep time: 20 mins | Servings: 12

Ingredients:

- 12 sheets Rice paper
- 12 leave Bib lettuce
- 12 Basil leaves
- ¾ c. Cilantro
- 1 shredded Carrot
- ½ sliced Cucumber
- 200 oz. cooked Shrimp

Directions:

1. Add all your vegetables, and shrimp to separate bowls and lay out on a flat surface. Set a damp paper towel tower flat on your work surface.
2. Quickly wet one of your rice papers under warm water and lay on paper towel.
3. Top with 1 of each vegetable, and 4 pieces of shrimp, then roll your rice paper into a burrito – like roll.
4. Repeat until all your vegetables and shrimp has been used up.
5. Serve, and enjoy.

Nutritional Information:

Calories: 67 Protein 2.62g, Carbs 7.39g, Fat 2.97g.

Washington Apple Turkey Gyro

Prep time: 10 mins | Servings: 6

Ingredients:

- 1 tsp. vegetable oil
- 1 c. sliced onion
- 1 c. sliced Red pepper
- 1 c. sliced Green pepper
- 2 tbsps. Lemon juice
- ½ lbs. Cooked turkey
- 1 chopped Golden apple
- 16 whole wheat Pocket pita bread
- 8 tbsps. Plain yogurt

Directions:

1. Over medium heat, add oil to a skillet and heat.
2. Add peppers, onion, and lemon juice and sauté until cook.
3. Mix in turkey and apple and cook until turkey is properly cooked.
4. Remove from flame. Place some of the mixture in each pita.
5. Fill each pita with some of mixture; drizzle with yogurt.
6. Serve warm.

Nutritional Information:

Calories: 235 Protein 11g, Carbs 31g, Fats 8g.

Pizza in a Pita

Prep time: 6 mins | Servings: 2

Ingredients:

- 2 whole wheat Pita bread
- ½ c. Mozzarella cheese
- ¼ c. Pizza sauce
- Toppings of choice: onion, mushrooms, olives, bell pepper, artichoke hearts, etc.

Directions:

1. Heat oven to 350 degrees F.
2. Slice the pita bread halfway from the top and scoop in the pizza sauce, cheese, and any desired topping.
3. Use aluminum foil to wrap pita and bake until cheese melts; roughly about 7 – 10 mins.

Nutritional Information:

Calories: 174 Protein 12.2g, Carbs 18g, Fat 7g.

Heartfelt Tuna Melt

Prep time: 15 mins | Servings: 4

Ingredients:

- 6 oz. White tuna packed in water
- 1/3 c. Chopped celery
- ¼ c. Chopped onion
- ¼ c. Thousand island salad dressing
- 2 whole wheat English muffins
- 3 oz. grated Cheddar cheese
- Salt
- Black pepper

Directions:

1. Heat broiler.
2. In a container, combine tuna, onion, celery and salad dressing.
3. Season to taste with salt and pepper.
4. Toast the halves of the English muffin.
5. On baking tray, place split side up, place 1/4 of tuna mixture on each half.
6. Broil for 3 mins or until heat is penetrated.
7. Place cheese on top and return tray to broiler for a minute longer or until cheese is melted.

Nutritional Information:

Calories: 197 Protein 16g, Carbs 21g, Fat 6g.

Spinach, Mushroom and Mozzarella Wraps

Prep time: 15 mins | Servings: 2

Ingredients:

- 1 tbsp. Olive oil
- 2½ c. sliced mushrooms
- 1 tsp. Minced garlic
- 2 whole wheat tortillas
- ½ lb. Fresh spinach
- 1 diced Plum tomato
- ¼ c. shredded Mozzarella cheese

Directions:

1. Put oven to heat at 350 degrees F. Over high heat, heat 1 tbsp. olive oil in a sauté pan.
2. Add layer of garlic and mushroom. As mushroom sauté, leave the mushrooms alone – exercise some patience as they become red-brown – turn on second side and sauté until it turns a similar color.
3. Arrange layers of spinach, tomato, mozzarella and cooked mushrooms on each tortilla.
4. Roll and place seam-side down in a lightly greased oven proof dish.
5. Bake uncovered for about 10 mins until cheese is melted.
6. Slice each tortilla into quarters in a crosswise direction.
7. Serve warm or as desired.

Nutritional Information:

Calories: 616 Protein 22g, Carbs 116g, Fat 15g.

Apple-Swiss Panini

Prep time: 8 mins | Servings: 4

Ingredients:

- 8 slices Whole-grain bread
- ¼ c. Honey mustard
- 2 sliced Apples
- 6 oz. sliced Swiss cheese
- 1 c. Arugula leaves
- Cooking spray

Directions:

1. On medium flame, preheat panini press on medium heat. Just use a non-stick skillet if you don't have a panini press.
2. Spread lightly, honey mustard over each slice of bread evenly over each slice of bread.
3. Place layers of apple slices, arugula leaves, and cheese over 4 bread slices.
4. Use remaining bread slices to top each.
5. Coat panini press lightly with cooking spray.
6. Allow 3 to 5 mins to grill sandwiches or until cheese has melted and bread toasted.
7. Transfer from pan and cool slightly before serving.

Nutritional Information:

Calories: 367 Protein 24g, Carbs 56g, Fat 6g.

California Grilled Veggie Sandwich

Prep time: 15 mins | Servings: 4

Ingredients:

- 3 tbsps. Mayonnaise
- 3 minced garlic cloves
- 1 tbsp. Lemon juice
- 1/8 c. Olive oil
- 1 c. sliced red bell peppers
- 1 sliced Zucchini
- 1 sliced red onion
- 1 sliced Yellow squash
- 2 slices Focaccia bread
- ½ c. Feta cheese

Directions:

1. Mix in a small bowl, mayonnaise, minced garlic, and lemon juice.
2. Place in the refrigerator.
3. Heat grill for high heat.
4. Lightly grease both the grill and your vegetables.
5. Set zucchini and bell peppers closest to the middle of the grill; set squash and onion pieces around them.
6. Cook for 3 minutes on each side (total of 6 mins) transfer from grill and put aside briefly.
7. Coat cut sides of bread with mayonnaise mixture. Topped with sprinkled feta cheese. With cheese side up, place bread on the grill, and seal lid.
8. Grill for 2 to 3 minutes.
9. After bread is removed from gill, layer with vegetables.
10. Serve as open face sandwiches.

Nutritional Information:

Calories: 178 Protein 6g, Carbs 9g, Fat 14g.

Chicken, Apple, and Spinach Salad

Prep time: 10 mins | Servings: 4

Ingredients

- 4 c. Spinach
- 2 c. chopped Apple
- 2 c. chopped chicken Breast
- ½ c. sliced red Onion
- ¼ c. chopped Pecans
- ¾ c. Acai Dressing

Directions:

1. Set 4 salad bowls on the table and add spinach to each.
2. Add each of your remaining ingredients as layers on top of the greens.
3. Once satisfied, drizzle each bowl of salad with 3 tablespoons of dressing.

Nutritional Information:

Calories: 410 Protein 30g, Carbs 20g, Fat 25g.

Orange Pineapple Chicken

Prep time: 10 mins | Servings: 4

Ingredients:

- ¼ c. Brown sugar
- 1/3 c. Orange juice
- 1½ lbs. Chicken parts
- 8 oz. Pineapple chunks in juice
- ½ tsp. Nutmeg
- ½ c. Golden raisins

Directions:

1. Put all ingredients into a large Ziploc bag and combine.
2. Freeze overnight and remove the next day.
3. Thaw completely. Set slow cooker to high.
4. Add contents to bag and cook for 7 hours until thoroughly cooked.

Nutritional Information:

Calories: 240.4 Protein 3.7g, Carbs 47.4g, Fat 4.3g.

Coconut Shrimp

Prep time: 10 mins | Servings: 4

Ingredients:

- 1 lb. Shrimp
- ¼ c. Heavy Cream
- 1 tbsp. Lemon Juice
- ¼ c. crushed Chives
- 4 tbsps. Butter
- 1 medium sliced tomato
- ¼ c. Coconut water
- Salt
- Pepper
- Pecans

Directions:

1. Melt butter in skillet over medium heat.
2. Place shrimp in pan and sauté for one minute.
3. Take off burner and pour in Coconut water and add back to burner.
4. Allow to cook for a few minutes while tossing then remove the shrimp and set aside.
5. Place heavy cream and tomatoes in a saucepan, bring the heat to a medium until thickened, pour in lemon juice and season with salt and pepper.
6. Drop the shrimp back into the mixture and warm in sauce. Plate and sprinkle chives and pecans.

Nutritional Information:

Calories: 310 Protein 9g, Carbs 31g, Fat 16g.

Steamed Spinach

Prep time: 10 mins | Servings: 1

Ingredients:

- 1 tsp. Salt
- 2 oz. Vegetable Oil
- 2 oz. Onion
- 1 tsp. Scotch Bonnet Pepper
- 4 oz. sliced Carrot
- 1 bundle Spinach
- 1 tsp. Black Pepper
- 4 oz. tomato
- 1 oz. green Onion
- 1 tsp. Thyme
- 1 tsp. unsalted butter

Directions:

1. Add your oil, carrots, pepper, and onions to a skillet and sauté until soft (for about a minute).
2. Add Spinach to skillet and season with salt and pepper to taste.
3. Cover and allow to cook for another 3 minutes.
4. Add your remaining ingredients to your pot allow to cook until spinach is tender (about 3 minutes longer).

Nutritional Information:

Calories: 74 Protein 5. 33g, Carbs 6.81g, Fat 4.16g.

Cinnamon Sweet Potatoes

Prep time: 10 mins | Servings: 3

Ingredients:

- 3 sweet potatoes
- ½ tsp. cinnamon powder
- 1 sliced onion
- ½ tsp. black pepper
- ½ tsp. salt
- 2 tbsps. olive oil

Directions:

1. Heat oil in pan and sauté onion for 1-2 minutes. Set aside.
2. Now combine sweet potatoes with onion and season with salt, pepper and cinnamon powder.
3. Preheat oven at 355 degrees.
4. Transfer to serving dish and bake for 30-35 minutes.

Nutritional Information:

Calories: 145.3 Protein 1.7g, Carbs 35.2g, Fat 0.4g.

Chicken Santa Fe

Prep time: 5 mins | Servings: 2

Ingredients:

- 15 oz. Canned corn
- 6 chicken breasts
- 15 oz. Canned black beans
- 1 c. shredded Cheddar cheese
- 1 c. Salsa

Directions:

1. Set slow cooker on high.
2. Combine corn, half of salsa and beans in slow cooker.
3. Put in chicken and top with remaining salsa.
4. Cover pot and cook for 2 hours 55 min or until chicken is thoroughly cooked.
5. Top with cheese and cook for 5 minutes more or until cheese melts.

Nutritional Information:

Calories: 370 Protein 30g, Carbs 29g, Fat 15g.

Tomato Bisque

Prep time: 10 mins | Servings: 4

Ingredients:

- 28 oz. tomatoes
- 1 c. coconut cream
- 1 diced onion
- 1 tsp. ground pepper
- 4 c. chicken stock
- 1 bunch chopped celery
- ½ c. chopped basil
- 1 tbsp. olive oil
- Salt
- pepper

Directions:

1. Heat olive oil in large pot over medium-high heat, add onion, with celery and cook until tender.
2. Pour chicken stock and tomatoes in the pot, bring mixture to simmer and season with salt and pepper. Simmer for 30 minutes.
3. Turn off heat and allow the soup to cool down.
4. Puree in bullet in batches. Stir in heavy cream, basil, and Parmesan cheese. Strain using a fine sieve. Serve immediately.

Nutritional Information:

Calories: 140 Protein 3g, Carbs 17g, Fat 7g.

Kung Pao Shrimp

Prep time: 15 mins | Servings: 2

Ingredients:

- 2 tbsps. Oil
- 1 sliced Ginger
- ¼ c. Onion
- 10 Red Chilies
- 12 oz. Shrimp
- ¼ c. Roasted Peanuts
- 3 Scallion stalks
- Kung Pao Sauce
- 2 tbsps. Soy Sauce
- 2 tbsps. Sweet soy sauce
- ½ tsp. Cornstarch
- 4 tbsps. Water
- ½ tsp. Sesame Oil
- ¼ tsp. White Pepper
- ½ tsp. Apple Cider Vinegar
- ½ tsp. Sugar

Directions:

1. Mix ingredients for sauce together and put aside till needed.
2. Heat oil in a wok then add ginger and stir. Put in green pepper, onion, and chilies.
3. Until you smell the chilies then add peanuts and shrimp and stir.
4. Add Kung Pao when shrimp has almost cooked.
5. Stir frequently to avoid sticking. Cook until sauce thickens then add scallions. Remove from heat and serve hot.

Nutritional Information:

Calories: 346 Protein 14g, Carbs 34g, Fat 19g.

Banana Waffles

Prep time: 10 mins | Servings: 6

Ingredients:

- 3 eggs
- 1 c. all-purpose flour
- 3 tbsps. melted butter
- 1 c. whole-wheat flour
- 1 ½ c. milk
- 2 tsps. baking powder
- ½ tsp. salt
- 2 tbsps. honey
- 2 ripe bananas

Directions:

1. In a bowl combine the flours, salt and baking powder.
2. In a blender combine the milk, honey, melted butter, and bananas.
3. Process until smooth.
4. Fold the banana mix into the dry ingredients and continue stirring until smooth. Let the batter rest for 10 minutes and preheat the waffle iron.
5. Pour 1/3 cup batter on the iron and cook for 4 minutes.
6. Serve with fresh fruits.

Nutritional Information:

Calories: 197.5 Protein 7.9g, Carbs 37.9g, Fat 3.1g.

BBQ Baked Beans

Prep time: 10 mins | Servings: 3

Ingredients:

- 1 chopped Yellow Onion
- 5 minced Garlic Cloves
- 1 chopped Jalapeno
- ¼ lb. diced Potatoes
- 1 lb. Pinto
- 6 c. Water
- 1 c. BBQ Sauce
- ½ c. dark brown sugar
- 2 tbsps. Spicy Brown Mustard
- 2 tbsps. Adobe Sauce
- 2 tbsps. Tabasco Sauce
- 2 tsps. Salt
- 2 tsps. Pepper

Directions:

1. Set your Dutch oven to preheat on the top of the stove.
2. Add potatoes to the heated oven and allow to brown. At this point, add the jalapeno and onions then proceed to sauté until onions become soft.
3. Continue to sauté while you add the garlic. Continue for about a minute.
4. Pour in the beans, and water then cover and allow cooking on low to medium heat for an hour to soften the beans.
5. Add a bit of your preferred BBQ sauce along with the brown sugar, adobo sauce, Tabasco, mustard salt and pepper while stirring well.
6. Remove the cover and allow simmering until the sauce thickens and the beans become completely cooked.

Nutritional Information:

Calories: 210 Protein 8g,Carbs 41g, Fat 1.5g.

Lasagna

Prep time: 15 mins | Servings: 8

Ingredients:

- 3 c. shredded mozzarella cheese
- 1 c. cottage cheese
- ¾ lb. lasagna noodles
- 3 ½ c. water
- 8 oz. unsalted tomato sauce
- 6 oz. unsalted tomato paste
- ¾ tsp. garlic powder
- ¾ tsp. oregano
- 1½ tsp. dried basil
- 1 sliced onion
- 1 lb. extra-lean ground beef

Directions:

1. Lightly coat a 10-14 cooking pan with cooking spray. Also, preheat the oven to 325 degrees Fahrenheit.
2. Now, for the sauce, put a large saucepan on the stove and place the ground beef and onion in it and cook until the meet is golden brown.
3. Once brown, drain the pan and then add the water, tomato sauce, tomato paste, garlic powder, oregano, and basil and stir until it comes to a boil. Reduce the heat and simmer for 10 minutes
4. In the cooking pan, place a half cup of the mixture on the bottom of the pan.
5. On top of the mixture, place a layer of the uncooked lasagna noodles and then add another layer of the mixture, as well as a cup of mozzarella cheese and a third of a cup of cottage cheese.
6. Do the same for the remaining mixture.
7. Place aluminum foil on top of the lasagna and put it into the oven.
8. Bake the lasagna for an hour and fifteen minutes or until the cheese is brown
9. Let the lasagna cool before serving.

Nutritional Information:

Calories: 425 Carbs 42g, Fat 13g, protein 33g.

Beef Stew with Fennel and Shallots

Prep time: 10 mins | Servings: 6

Ingredients:

- 1/3 c. chopped fresh parsley
- 3 Portobello mushrooms
- 18 small boiling onions
- 4 large red-skinned potatoes
- 4 large sliced carrots
- 3 c. vegetable stock
- 1 bay leaf
- 2 fresh thyme sprigs
- ¾ tsp. ground black pepper
- 3 large shallots
- ½ fennel bulb
- 2 tbsps. olive oil
- 1 lb. boneless lean beef stew meat
- 3 tbsps. all- purpose flour

Directions:

1. Start by placing the flour on a place and rolling the beef cubes in the flour
2. Then, using a large saucepan, pour the oil in and heat at medium heat.
3. Once the beef is floured, put it into the sauce pan and cook until brown on all sides.
4. Remove the beef and let cook elsewhere.
5. Without changing the temperature, place the shallots and the fennel in the pan and cook until they are a light brown.
6. Add the lay leaf, thyme sprigs, and a quarter of the pepper to the mix and let cook for a minute or two.
7. Now, add the beef back into the pan with the vegetable stock and bring the mixture to a boil. After, reduce the heat and cover it while it simmers. Leave it like this for 45 minutes.
8. Once the meat is tender, add the mushrooms, onions, potatoes, and carrots.
9. Stir the mixture and let simmer for another 30 minutes.
10. Pull the bay leaf and the thyme sprigs out of the stew and stir in the parsley and remaining pepper.
11. Serve immediately.

Nutritional Information:

Calories: 244 Fat 8g, Carbs 22g, protein 21g.

Grilled Portobello Mushroom Burger

Prep time: 15 mins | Servings: 4

Ingredients:

- 2 romaine lettuce leaves
- 4 slices of red onion
- 1 slices of tomato
- 4 whole-wheat toasted buns
- 2 tbsp. olive oil
- ¼ tsp. cayenne pepper
- 1 minced garlic clove
- 1 tbsp. sugar
- ½ c. water
- 1/3 c. balsamic vinegar
- 4 large Portobello mushroom caps

Directions:

1. The Portobello mushrooms need to be cleaned and their stems need to be removed and the caps need to be set aside.
2. Now, in a small bowl the olive oil, cayenne pepper, garlic, sugar, water, and vinegar need to be mixed together and pored over top the mushroom caps.
3. The caps need to be placed into a plastic container, covered, and placed into the refrigerator to marinate for an hour.
4. Turn on the grill and lightly coat it in cooking spray—or, turn on the stove and coat a frying pan in the same substance.
5. Fry or grill the mushrooms on medium heat, making sure to flip them often. Usually, it will take five minutes on each side.
6. Place the mushrooms on their own bun and top with half a lettuce leaf, one onion slice and one tomato slice.
7. Serve immediately.

Nutritional Information:

Calories: 301 Fat 9g, Carbs 45g, protein 10g.

Chicken Brats

Prep time: 10 mins | Servings: 6

Ingredients:

- 1 tsp. celery seed
- 1 tsp. ground mustard seed
- ¼ tsp. nutmeg
- 1 tsp. minced rosemary
- ½ tsp. cayenne pepper
- ½ tsp. white pepper
- 1 tsp. black pepper
- 1 tsp. paprika
- 1 tsp. cumin seed
- 2 tsps. fennel seed
- 1 lb. ground chicken breast
- 1 c. cooked brown rice
- ½ tsp. canola oil
- 4 minced garlic
- 1 c. minced yellow onion

Ingredients:

1. In a frying pan, sauté the canola oil, garlic, and onion until golden.
2. Place the browned onion and garlic in the cooked rice and mix in all the other herbs and spices with the ground chicken breast.
3. Let the mixture marinate in the fridge for about an hour.
4. Pre-heat the oven to 350 degrees Fahrenheit.
5. Remove from the fridge and roll the mixture into sausage shapes and place on a cooking sheet.
6. Bake in the oven for about 5-10 minutes, or until cooked.
7. Let the sausages cool before serving.

Nutritional Information:
Calories: 156 ,Fat 4g, Carbs 12g, protein 18g.

Asian Pork Tenderloin

Prep time: 20 mins | Servings: 4

Ingredients:

- 1 lb. pork tenderloin
- 1 tbsp. sesame seed oil
- 1/8 tsp. ground cinnamon
- ¼ tsp. ground cumin
- ½ tsp. celery seed
- 1/8 tsp. cayenne pepper
- 1 tsp. ground coriander
- 2 tbsps. sesame seeds

Directions:

1. Preheat the oven to four hundred degrees Fahrenheit.
2. While the oven is preheating, grease a baking sheet with cooking spray.
3. Pull out a frying pan and on low heat fry the sesame seeds while stirring contently.
4. After one to two minutes, or the sesame seeds are golden brown, remove the seeds from the heat and set them aside.
5. In a large mixing bowl, place the toasted sesame seeds, sesame seed oil, cinnamon, cumin, celery seed, cayenne pepper, and coriander inside and stir until it is mixed evenly.
6. Using the prepared baking dish, place the tenderloin on top and evenly space them out.
7. Use a brush to lather the tenderloin, on both sides, with the mixture.
8. Place the baking sheet inside the oven and let bake for about fifteen minutes or until they are no longer pink. Take the tenderloin out and serve with a side dish immediately.

Nutritional Information:

Calories: 248 Carbs 1g, Fat 16g, protein 26g

White Chicken Chili

Prep time: 10 mins | Servings: 8

Ingredients:

- 3 tbsps. chopped cilantro
- 8 tbsps. shredded Monterey jack cheese
- 1 tsp. cayenne pepper
- 1 tsp. dried oregano
- 1 tsp. ground cumin
- 2 tsps. chili powder
- 2 minced garlic cloves
- 1 sliced red pepper
- ½ sliced green pepper
- 4 c. low-sodium chicken broth
- 1 can diced tomatoes
- 2 cans white beans
- 1 can white chunk chicken

Directions:

1. Grab a large cooking pot and place the chicken broth, tomatoes, and chicken inside.
2. Bring the mixture to a boil and then cover it to let it simmer.
3. While the mixture is simmering, take a non-stick frying pan, cover it in cooking spray, and add the garlic, peppers, and onions.
4. Fry the vegetables until golden brown or to your liking.
5. Add the contents of the frying pan to the cooking pot.
6. Add the cayenne pepper, oregano, cumin, and chili powder and cover the mixture again.
7. Raise the heat up to medium and let it simmer for about ten more minutes.
8. Ladle the chili into bowls and serve immediately.
9. Use cilantro only as a garnish.

Nutritional Information:

Calories: 212 ,Fat 4g, Carbs 25g, protein 19g.

Brown Stewed Fish

Prep time: 10 mins | Servings: 4

Ingredients:

- 2 lbs. fish
- 1 diced large onion
- 2 small tomatoes
- 3 stalks scallion
- 1 c. vegetables
- ¾ c. fish stock
- 2 slices hot pepper
- 1 tsp. salt
- ¼ c. oil

Directions:

1. Scale, clean and prepare fish for frying.
2. Allow oil to cool, strain nearly all of it from frying pan, put aside.
3. Sauté seasonings and vegetables in frying pan.
4. Add water or stock to frying pan with sautéed vegetables and simmer until all flavors blend.
5. Add fish, cover and cook for five minutes.

Nutritional Information:

Calories: 352 ,Protein 31.6g, Carbs 11.4g, Fat 19.7g.

Grilled Cod

Prep time: 15 mins | Servings: 2

Ingredients:

- 2 cod fillets
- ½ tsp. garlic paste
- 3 tbsps. lemon juice
- 1 tsp. salt
- ½ tsp. black pepper
- ½ tsp. oregano
- 1 tsp. fish sauce
- ¼ tsp. turmeric powder
- 2 tbsps. olive oil

Directions:

1. Sprinkle turmeric powder on fish and rub all over.
2. Leave it for 10-15 minutes then wash out fish well.
3. Take a bowl add vinegar, lemon juice, pepper, salt, fish sauce and oregano, toss to combine.
4. Spread this mixture on fish fillets and rub on it with hands.

Nutritional Information:

Calories: 138 ,Protein 23.71g, Carbs 0.46g, Fat 4.07g.

Baked Salmon

Prep time: 10 mins | Servings: 6

Ingredients:

- 1½ lbs. salmon fillets
- ½ sliced onion
- 1 c. chopped grape tomatoes
- 1 tsp. dried basil
- 1 tbsp. chopped chives
- 1 tsp. dried rosemary
- 1 tsp. garlic powder
- 1 tsp. salt
- 1/3 c. soy sauce
- 1/3 c. brown sugar
- 1/3 c. water
- ¼ c. vegetable oil

Directions:

1. Preheat oven to 350 degrees F.
2. Season salmon fillets with onion, basil, rosemary, garlic powder, and salt.
3. In a small bowl, combine brown sugar, soy sauce, water, and vegetable oil until sugar is dissolved.
4. Place fillets in a Ziploc bag or airtight container with soy sauce mixture and place in refrigerator for 2 hours to marinate.
5. Preheat grill at medium heat. Lightly oil grill grate. Place fillets on the preheated grill and cook for 6 to 8 minutes per side.

Nutritional Information:

Calories: 274 Protein 24g, Carbs 1g, Fat 19g.

Steamed Mussels

Prep time: 5 mins | Servings: 4

Ingredients:

- 6 oz. chorizo
- 1 c. white wine
- 2 tbsps. olive oil
- 1 sliced onion
- 4 lbs. mussels
- 3 sprigs thyme
- 1 tsp. smoked paprika
- 14.5 oz. diced tomatoes
- 4 sliced garlic cloves
- Salt
- pepper

Directions:

1. over medium heat, warm olive oil.
2. Add the onion, season to taste and cook until softened for 3-4 minutes.
3. Add garlic and cook for an additional 1 minute.
4. Stir in the smoked paprika and cook for 30 seconds or until fragrant.
5. Add the chorizo, wine, and tomatoes.
6. Add the fresh thyme and bring to a simmer.
7. Stir in the mussels and coat with sauce.
8. Cover and cook until mussels are opened.
9. Discard all unopened ones.
10. Serve mussels while still hot with toasted bread slices.

Nutritional Information:

Calories: 256 Protein 35.4g, Carbs 10.98g, Fat 6.66g.

Saucy Chicken

Prep time: 15 mins | Servings: 4

Ingredients:

- 8 chicken tights
- 1 c. chicken broth
- 1 tbsp. sherry vinegar
- 1½ c. roasted red peppers, chopped
- 4 crushed garlic cloves
- 1½ c. diced russet potatoes
- 2 tsps. chopped thyme leaves

Directions:

1. Preheat oven to 425F.
2. Heat olive oil in a pan over medium-high heat.
3. Season the chicken tights with salt and pepper and place into heated oil, skin side down. Cook the chicken without moving around for 3 minutes or until browned. Transfer to a plate and repeat with remaining chicken.
4. Add the garlic and thyme to the same skillet. Cook until fragrant.
5. Add the potatoes, chicken broth, red peppers, and vinegar to the pan.
6. Bring to boil and once boils remove from the heat.
7. Return the chicken to the pan, skin side up and place in the oven.
8. Braise the chicken for 30 minutes or until the potatoes are tender.
9. Serve while still hot with baguette or some other bread.

Nutritional Information:

Calories: 125.5 Protein 11.7g,Carbs 16.7g, Fat 1.6g.

Chicken Fried Rice

Prep time: 6 mins | Servings: 2

Ingredients:

- 2 tbsps. Oil
- 2 minced garlic cloves
- 4 oz. cubed chicken breast
- 4 oz. Shrimp
- 1 c. Mix vegetables- frozen
- 12 oz. Overnight rice
- 1 tbsp. Fish Sauce
- 1 tbsp. Soy Sauce
- ¼ tsp. Oyster Sauce
- ¼ tsp. White Pepper
- 2 Eggs
- ¼ tsp. Salt

Directions:

1. In a pan, add oil and garlic, cook, until the aroma of the garlic becomes present.
2. Add shrimp, chicken, and vegetables.
3. Put in in rice and stir to combine with veggies.
4. Add soy sauce, fish sauce, oyster sauce, salt, and pepper and stir the rice for a few minutes.
5. Use a spatula to make a gap in the center of the rice.
6. Dispense eggs in the center and let it sit for 30 seconds.
7. Use rice to cover eggs and stir as egg cooks.
8. Add some salt and stir a bit more then serve.

Nutritional Information:

Calories: 309.6 Protein 15g, Carbs 50g, Fat 5g.

Buffalo & Ranch Chicken Meatloaf

Prep time: 10 mins | Servings: 6

Ingredients:

- ½ c. Ranch Dressing
- ¼ c. Buffalo Wing Sauce
- 675g Ground Chicken
- 120g Chicken Stuffing Mix
- ½ c. Feta Cheese
- 1 sliced celery stalk
- 2 chopped green Onion
- 1 Egg

Directions:

1. Preheat oven to 375 degrees and lightly grease a 6 x 4-inch loaf tin with olive oil.
2. Mix all your egg and dry ingredients, along with half of your dressing ingredients together until fully incorporated using your hands.
3. Once combined, add your meat mixture into your greased loaf tin, top with the other half of your dressing ingredients and set to bake until done (about 30 to 35 minutes).
4. Tip: Use a thermometer to determine doneness by inserting it into the thickest part of the meatloaf. Ensure it reads 165 degrees F.

Nutritional Information:

Calories: 119 Protein 6g, Carbs 14g, Fat 4g.

Shitake & Snow Peas Quinoa

Prep time: 10 mins | Servings: 4

Ingredients:

- 3 c. Fluffy Quinoa
- 1 tbsp. Sesame Oil
- 1 tbsp. Garlic Cloves
- 4 oz. Shitake Mushroom
- 4 oz. Snow Peas
- ¼ tsp. Salt
- ¼ tsp. Pepper
- 1 tbsp. Soy Sauce
- 1 sliced green Onion

Directions:

1. In a medium non-stick skillet heat your sesame oil on medium heat.
2. Add your garlic and allow to cook for about a minute stirring frequently so that it doesn't burn.
3. Add in your mushrooms and cook until tender (should be about 5 min)
4. Next, add the snow peas, salt, and pepper. Then continue stirring until peas become bright green in color (it generally takes about 3 minutes) then remove from the heat.
5. Now, add in all the remaining ingredients and toss until fully combined.
6. Serve and enjoy.

Nutritional Information:

Calories: 210 Protein 8g, Carbs 32g, Fat 6g.

Chili Chicken Curry

Prep time: 5 mins | Servings: 4

Ingredients:

- 14 oz. kidney beans
- 3 tbsp. red curry paste
- 1 lb. ground chicken
- 1 tbsp. tomato paste
- 12 oz. black beans
- 1 tbsp. chili powder
- 2 tsp. dried oregano
- 1 c. tomato sauce
- Vegetable oil
- 1 tsp. Salt
- 1 tsp. Pepper

Directions:

1. Heat the oil in a rice cooker.
2. Add curry paste and stir.
3. Place the chicken into a heated rice cooker.
4. Cook until cooked thoroughly. Once cooked add the beans, tomato paste, and sauce.
5. Stir and add the spices. Serve.

Nutritional Information:

Calories: 313.5 Protein 31.9g, Carbs 25.5g, Fat 9g.

Baked Pumpkin Pasta

Prep time: 10 mins | Servings: 4

Ingredients:

- 1 c. boneless chicken
- 1 c. pumpkin
- 1 package pasta
- ½ tsp. garlic paste
- 1 chopped onion
- 1 tsp. black pepper
- ½ tsp. salt
- 2 tbsps. olive oil
- 1 c. cheddar cheese

Directions:

1. Preheat oven at 355 degrees.
2. Heat oil in pan and sauté onion with garlic for 1 minute.
3. Add pumpkin and cook for 3-4 minutes. Season with salt and pepper.
4. Now add chicken pieces and stir for 1 minute.

Nutritional Information:

Calories:307 Protein 17.7g, Carbs 51.5g, Fat 3.8g.

Gruyere and Spinach Casserole

Prep time: 10 mins | Servings: 5

Ingredients:

- 2 c. chopped spinach
- 2 eggs
- 1 tsp. sugar
- 2 oz. grated gruyere
- 1 c. grated parmesan cheese
- ¼ tsp. salt
- ½ c. chopped green onion
- 4 minced garlic cloves
- 2 eggs
- 1 tsp. chili powder
- 1 c. heavy milk
- 2 tbsps. olive oil

Directions:

1. Heat oil in saucepan and sauté garlic for 1 minute with onion.
2. Add spinach and stir for 2-3 minutes till its color is lightly changed.
3. In separate bowl add eggs and whisks for 1-2 minutes. Add in milk, gruyere and whisk again for 1 minute.
4. Transfer this mixture in spinach mixture and cook for 2 minutes.
5. Season with salt and chili powder.
6. Preheat oven at 355 degrees. Add gruyere mixture in baking dish, top with parmesan cheese and bake for 40-45 minutes.
7. Serve and enjoy.

Nutritional Information:

Calories: 270 ,Protein 18g, Carbs 8g, Fat 19g.

Prep time: 15 mins | Servings: 6

Ingredients:

- 1 whole turkey
- 2 tsps. garlic paste
- 1 tsp. ginger powder
- 2 tablespoons soya sauce
- 1 tsp. cayenne pepper
- 1 tsp. salt
- ½ tsp. black pepper
- 3 tbsps. lemon juice
- 2 tbsps. red wine vinegar
- ½ tsp. mustard powder
- 1 tsp. cinnamon powder
- 2 tbsps. sesame seeds oil

Directions:

1. In a bowl add garlic paste, ginger powder, cayenne pepper, black pepper, cinnamon powder, mustard powder, lemon juice, oil, vinegar, soya sauce and salt, mix well.
2. Now pour this marinate over turkey and rub with hands all over it.
3. Cover and leave to marinade for 15-20 minutes. Preheat oven at 355 degrees.
4. Spread aluminum foil in baking tray and place turkey on it.
5. Bake for 40-45 minutes or till nicely golden.
6. Serve and enjoy.

Nutritional Information:

Calories: 240.4 , 3.7g, Protein 47.4g, Carbs 4.3g, Fat

Honey Garlic Chicken Drumsticks

Prep time: 15 mins | Servings: 6

Ingredients:

- 8 chicken drumsticks
- 3 tsps. garlic powder
- 1 tsp. ginger powder
- 3 tbsps. soya sauce
- 1 tsp. cayenne pepper
- 1 tsp. salt
- 2 tbsps. Barbecue sauce
- 2 tbsps. lime juice
- ¼ c. apple cider vinegar
- 2 tbsps. olive oil
- 3 tbsps. honey

Directions:

1. In a bowl add ginger powder, garlic powder, soya sauce, honey, vinegar, lime juice, barbecue sauce, salt, pepper and toss to combine.
2. Add in chicken drumsticks and mix well, leave to marinade for 20 minutes. Preheat oven at 355 degrees.
3. Transfer drumsticks in baking tray and bake for 30-35 minutes or till golden brown.
4. Serve and enjoy.

Nutritional Information:

Calories: 121.2 ,Protein 8.1g, Carbs 15.5g, Fat 3.3g.

Shrimp Pasta Primavera

Prep time: 15 mins | Servings: 6

Ingredients:

- 1¼ c. sliced Asparagus
- 12 oz. whole wheat Penne
- 1 c. Green peas
- 2 tsps. Olive oil
- 1 tbsp. minced Garlic
- 1/8 tsp. crushed Red pepper
- 1 lb. Shrimp
- ½ c. sliced green onion
- 2 tsps. Lemon juice
- 1 tbsp. chopped Parsley
- 1/3 c. grated Parmesan cheese
- ½ tsp. Salt
- ½ tsp. Pepper

Directions:

1. Set a large saucepan over high heat, and allow to come to a boil.
2. Once boiling, add asparagus then cook until fork tender (about 4 minutes). Carefully remove the asparagus from the hot water using a slotted spoon then add your pasta to the same pot.
3. Cook until done based on the instructions on the package. When the pasta was 2 minutes out add peas.
4. When fully cooked, drain, and add to a large bowl with the asparagus. Next, set a skillet with olive oil over medium heat, then add red pepper, and garlic, then cook, while stirring for about a minute.
5. Add shrimp and cook until it becomes opaque (about 4 minutes, stirring).
6. Add your remaining ingredients to the skillet on top of shrimp and toss to coat.

Nutritional Information:

Calories: 440 Protein 31g Carbs 31g, Fat 18g.

Easy Shrimp Salad

Prep time: 10 mins | Servings: 6

Ingredients:

For the shrimp:

- 2 minced garlic cloves
- 1 lb. shrimp
- 1 tsp. Cajun spice
- 2 tbsps. olive oil

For the salad:

- 6 c. lettuce leaves
- 4 chopped tomatoes
- 1 chopped yellow onion
- 1 sliced cucumber
- 2 chopped avocados

- 1 c. corn
- 1 lemon
- ½ bunch chopped parsley
- 2 tbsps. olive oil
- Black pepper

Directions:

1. In a bowl, combine the shrimp with Cajun spice and garlic and toss.
2. Heat up a pan with 2 tablespoons oil over medium-high heat, add shrimp, cook each side for 2 minutes and set to a bowl.
3. Add lettuce, tomatoes, onion, cucumber, avocado, corn and a pinch of pepper and toss.
4. In a small bowl, mix 2 tablespoons oil with parsley and lemon juice, whisk well, pour over the salad, toss and serve for lunch.

Nutritional Information:

Calories: 210 Fat 4g, Carbs 28g, protein 14g.

Easy Veggie Soup

Prep time: 10 mins | Servings: 6

Ingredients:

- 1 tbsp. olive oil
- 1 chopped yellow onion
- 2 chopped celery ribs
- 2 chopped carrots
- 2 c. mixed zucchini and cauliflower florets
- black pepper
- 1 tsp. dried thyme
- ½ tsp. garlic powder
- 1 tsp. dried oregano
- 8 c. veggie stock
- 1 bay leaf
- 14 oz. chopped canned tomatoes

Directions:

1. Add oil in a pot and heat over medium-high heat, add onion, celery and carrots, stir and sauté them for 4 minutes.
2. Add zucchini, cauliflower, black pepper, thyme, garlic powder, oregano, bay leaf, tomatoes and stock, stir, bring to a simmer and cook for 16 minutes.
3. Stir the soup one more time, ladle it into bowls and serve for a dash diet lunch. Enjoy!

Nutritional Information:

Calories: 180 Fat 2g, Carbs 28g, protein 8g .

Seafood Salad

Prep time: 15 mins | Servings: 4

Ingredients:

- 1 big octopus
- 1 lb. mussels
- 2 lbs. clams
- 1 big squid
- 3 chopped garlic cloves
- 1 celery rib
- ½ c. sliced celery rib
- 1 carrot
- 1 chopped white onion
-
- 1 bay leaf
- ¾ c. veggie stock
- 2 c. sliced radicchio
- 1 sliced red onion
- 1 c. chopped parsley
- 1 c. olive oil
- 1 c. red wine vinegar
- Black pepper

1. Place the octopus in a large pot with celery rib cut into thirds, garlic, carrot, bay leaf, white onion and stock. Add water to cover the octopus, cover the pot, bring to a boil over high heat, and reduce temperature to low, simmer for 1 hour and 30 minutes. Drain octopus, reserve boiling liquid and leave it aside to cool down.
2. Put ¼ cup octopus cooking liquid in another pot, add mussels, heat up over medium-high heat, cook until they open, transfer to a bowl and leave aside.
3. Add clams to the pan, cover, cook over medium-high heat until they open as well, transfer to the bowl with mussels and leave aside.
4. Add squid to the pan, cover and cook over medium-high heat for 3 minutes, transfer to the bowl with mussels and clams.
5. Meanwhile, slice octopus into small pieces and mix with the rest of the seafood.
6. Add sliced celery, radicchio, red onion, vinegar, olive oil, parsley, salt and pepper, toss and leave aside in the fridge for 2 hours before serving. Enjoy!

Nutritional Information:

Calories: 200 Fat 8g, carbs 28g, protein 4g

Caesar Salad

Prep time: 10 mins | Servings: 4

Ingredients:

- 1 lb. chicken breast
- Cooking spray
- Black pepper
- ½ c. cubed feta cheese
- 2 tbsps. lemon juice
- 1½ tsps. Dijon mustard
- 1 tbsp. olive oil
- 1½ tsps. red wine vinegar
- ¾ tsp. minced garlic
- 1 tbsp. water
- 1 tsp. Worcestershire sauce
- 8 c. lettuce leaves
- 4 tbsps. grated parmesan
- 1¼ whole wheat croutons

Directions:

1. Spray chicken breasts with some cooking spray and season black pepper to the taste.
2. Heat up your kitchen grill over medium-high heat, add chicken breasts, cook for 6 minutes on each side, transfer to a cutting board, cool down for a few minutes, cut in small pieces, transfer to a salad bowl, add lettuce and croutons and leave aside.

3. In your blender, mix feta with lemon juice, olive oil, mustard, vinegar, Worcestershire sauce and garlic and pulse well.
4. Add the water and half of the parmesan and blend some more.
5. Add this to your salad, toss to coat, sprinkle the rest of the parmesan and serve.

Nutritional Information:
Calories: 200 Fat 10g, Carbs 18g, protein 10g.

Greek Chicken Salad

Prep time: 10 minutes | Servings: 4

Ingredients:
- 15 oz. canned chickpeas
- 9 oz. chicken breast
- 1 chopped cucumber
- 4 chopped green onions
- Black pepper
- ½ c. yoghurt
-

- ¼ c. chopped mint
- 2 c. baby spinach
- 2 minced garlic cloves
- 1/3 c. feta cheese
- 4 lemon wedges

Directions:
1. In a salad bowl, mix chicken meat with chickpeas, cucumber, onions, mint, garlic, salt and pepper.
2. Add yogurt, spinach and feta and toss to coat.
3. Serve with lemon wedges on the side.
4. Enjoy!

Nutritional Information:
Calories: 180 Fat 10g, Carbs 16g, protein 10g.

Chicken Soup

Prep time: 10 mins | Servings: 6

Ingredients:
- 1 whole chicken
- 6 chopped celery stalks
- 6 sliced carrots

- 1 onion
- 1 bunch parsley springs
- 1 bunch dill springs

- 2 tbsps. chopped dill
- 3 garlic cloves
- 2 tbsps. black peppercorns
- black pepper
- 2 bay leaves
- ¼ tsp. saffron threads

Directions:

1. Put chicken pieces in a pot, add water to cover, bring to a boil over medium-high heat, cook for 15 minutes and skim foam.
2. Add celery, onion, carrots, parsley springs, dill springs, whole cloves, bay leaves, peppercorns and some black pepper, stir, cover pot, reduce heat to medium-low and simmer for 1 hour and 30 minutes.
3. Take chicken pieces out and leave them aside to cool down.
4. Strain soup into another pot, reserve carrots and celery but discard herbs and spices.
5. Discard bones from the chicken, cut meat into strips and return to pot.
6. Heat up the soup with reserved veggies, add chicken pieces, crushed saffron and chopped dill and stir.
7. Ladle soup into bowls and serve. Enjoy!

Nutritional Information:
Calories: 200 Fat 10g, Carbs 16g, protein 12g.

Pumpkin Soup

Prep time: 10 mins | Servings: 4

Ingredients:

- 1 chopped yellow onion
- ¾ c. water
- 15 oz. pumpkin puree
- 2 c. veggie stock
- ½ tsp. cinnamon powder
- ¼ tsp. ground nutmeg
- 1 c. fat-free milk
- Black pepper
- 1 chopped green onion

Directions:

1. Put the water in a pot, bring to a simmer over medium heat, add onion, stock and pumpkin puree and stir.
2. Add cinnamon, nutmeg, milk and black pepper, stir, cook for 10 minutes, ladle into bowls, sprinkle green onion on top and serve.
3. Enjoy!

Nutritional Information:
Calories: 180 Fat 10g, Carbs 22g, protein 14g.

Spicy Black Bean Soup

Prep time: 10 mins | Servings: 8

Ingredients:

- 1 lb. black beans
- 2 chopped yellow onions
- 2 quarts low-sodium veggie stock
- 2 tbsps. olive oil
- 6 minced garlic cloves
- 2 chopped tomatoes
- 2 chopped jalapenos
- ½ tsp. dried oregano
- 1 tsp. ground cumin
- 1 tsp. grated ginger
- 2 bay leaves
- 1 tbsp. chili powder
- 3 tbsps. balsamic vinegar
- Black pepper
- ½ c. chopped scallions

Directions:

1. Put the stock in a pot, bring to a simmer over medium heat, add beans, cover and cook for 45 minutes.
2. Meanwhile, heat up a pan with the oil over medium-high heat, add ginger, garlic and onion, stir and cook for 5 minutes.
3. Add tomatoes, cumin, jalapeno, oregano and chili powder, stir, cook for 3 minutes more and transfer to the pot with the beans.
4. Add bay leaves, and cook the soup for 40 minutes more while the pot is covered.
5. Add vinegar, stir, cook the soup for 15 minutes more, discard bay leaves, blend the soup using an immersion blender, ladle into bowls and serve with scallions on top. Enjoy!

Nutritional Information:
Calories: 220, fat 10, carbs 34, protein 14

Shrimp Soup

Prep time: 10 mins | Servings: 6

Ingredients:

- 8 oz. shrimp
- 1 stalk lemongrass
- 2 grated ginger
- 6 c. low-sodium chicken stock
- 2 chopped jalapenos
- 4 lime leaves
- 1½ c. chopped pineapple
- 1 c. chopped shiitake mushroom caps
- 1 chopped tomato
- ½ cubed bell pepper
- 1 tsp. stevia

- ¼ c. lime juice
- 1/3 c. chopped cilantro
- 2 sliced scallions

Directions:

1. In a pot, mix ginger with lemongrass, stock, jalapenos and lime leaves, stir, bring to a boil over medium heat, cover, cook for 15 minutes, strain liquid in a bowl and discard solids.
2. Return soup to the pot again, add pineapple, tomato, mushrooms, bell pepper, sugar and fish sauce, stir, bring to a boil over medium heat, cook for 5 minutes, add shrimp and cook for 3 more minutes.
3. Add lime juice, cilantro and scallions, stir, ladle into soup bowls and serve.
4. Enjoy!

Nutritional Information:

Calories: 190 Fat 8g, Carbs 30g, protein 6g.

Mayo-less Tuna Salad

Prep time: 5 mins | Servings: 2

Ingredients:

- 5 oz. Tuna
- 1 tbsp. extra virgin Olive oil
- 1 tbsp. Red wine vinegar
- ¼ c. chopped green onion
- 2 c. Arugula
- 1 c. cooked Pasta
- 1 tbsp. Parmesan cheese
- Black pepper

Directions:

1. Combine all your ingredients into a medium bowl.
2. Split mixture between two plates.
3. Serve, and enjoy.

Nutritional Information:

Calories: 213.2 Protein 22.7g, Carbs 20.3g, Fat 6.2g,

Chestnut Soup

Prep time: 10 mins | Servings: 3

Ingredients:

- 30 oz. whole roasted chestnuts
- 1 chopped shallot
- ½ c. heavy cream
- ½ c. chicken stock
- 1 chopped leek
- 2 tbsps. butter
- 1 sprig thyme
- 1 bay leaf
- 1 chopped celery stalk
- ½ tsp. nutmeg
- Salt
- pepper

Directions:

1. Add butter, carrot, leek, shallot, and celery in a saucepan over medium heat. Cook for 6-7 minutes or until the vegetables are tender.
2. Add stock, thyme, bay leaf, chestnuts and bring to boil. Reduce heat and simmer for 25 minutes.
3. Remove from the heat and discard the thyme and bay leaf.
4. Allow to cool slightly and puree using an immersion blender.
5. Heat the soup again as you stir in the cream, nutmeg and season to taste.
6. Cook for 5 minutes more.
7. Serve while still hot.

Nutritional Information:

Calories: 191 Protein 6g, Carbs 25g, Fat 18g.

Pepper Pot Soup

Prep time: 10 mins | Servings: 6

Ingredients:

- 4 quarts chicken stock
- 3 tbsps. butter
- 2 diced potatoes
- ½ diced breadfruit
- 1 lb. diced yam
- ½ lb. diced cocoa
- 2 crushed garlic cloves
- 2 sprigs thyme
- 1 scotch bonnet
- 3 chopped green onion
- ½ c. Coconut Milk
- 10 pimento berries
- 2 chopped callaloo

Directions:

1. In a reasonable size soup pot, boil 4 quarts of stock.
2. Add garlic, potato, breadfruit, yam, cocoa, and stir.
3. Bring soup to a boil add thyme, green onion, pimento, callaloo, coconut milk, and pepper.
4. Stir, and cook until done.

Nutritional Information:

Calories: 250.3 Protein 15.5g, Carbs 22.8g, Fat 11.3g.

Quinoa & Avocado Salad

Prep time: 10 mins | Servings: 2

Ingredients:

- 1½ c. Cooked Quinoa
- 4 oz. julienned Cucumber
- 4 oz. julienned Carrots
- ½ diced Avocado
- ½ c. Brussels Sprouts

Directions:

1. Split your Quinoa into 2 medium bowls.
2. Mix in your minced nori.
3. Top with your cucumber, avocado, and carrot.
4. Add blanched Brussel Sprouts.
5. Serve and enjoy!

Nutritional Information:

Calories: 472 Protein 11.2g, Carbs 50.6g, Fat 27.4g.

Kale Salad with Mixed Vegetables

Prep time: 10 mins | Servings: 4

Ingredients:

- 1 bunch chopped Premier kale
- 1 c. fresh peas
- 2 chopped carrots
- 1 c. boiled potatoes
- 1 c. sliced cabbage
- 2 tbsps. apple cider vinegar
- 1 tsp. chili powder
- ½ tsp. salt
- 2 tbsps. coconut oil
- 1 tsp. coconut powder

Directions:

1. Combine all vegetables with kale.
2. Drizzle vinegar and coconut oil.
3. Season with salt and chili powder.
4. Sprinkle coconut powder and toss to combine.
5. Add to a serving dish and serve. Enjoy.

Nutritional Information:

Calories: 240 Protein 9g, Carbs 36g, Fat 9g.

Cream of Corn Soup

Prep time: 15 mins | Servings: 4

Ingredients:

- 0.5 lb. Corn puree
- 0.5 lb. carrots
- 2 c. vegetable stock
- ½ c. chopped onion
- ½ tsp. Salt
- ¼ tsp. Pepper
- 1 tsp. dried thyme
- 2 oz. chopped celery
- ½ tbsp. olive oil
- 1 anise star

Directions:

1. Heat olive oil in medium pot and add onion; add celery, carrots and sauté for 15 minutes, until onion is caramelized.
2. Add corn and stir until corn is tender.

3. Add thyme and stir well.
4. Transfer the vegetables in a blender, add pumpkin puree, vegetable stock, and pulse until smooth.
5. Transfer the mixture into sauce pan and simmer, add anise star and simmer over medium-high heat for 5-8 minutes or until heated through.
6. Remove the anise star and discard.
7. Serve immediately.

Nutritional Information:

Calories: 223 Protein 7.84g, Carbs 23.98g, Fat 11.51g.

Clam Soup

Prep time: 15 mins | Servings: 4

Ingredients:

- 1½ c. Water
- ½ fresh ginger
- 1 lb. Manila clams
- 1 tbsp. Chinese rice white wine
- ¼ tsp. Salt
- ¼ tsp. White Pepper

Directions:

1. In a large pot, boil water and add clams and ginger.
2. Cook until clams open then add wine.
3. Add pepper and salt and serve hot.

Nutritional Information:

Calories: 80 Protein 3g, Carbs 16g, Fat 0.5g.

Apple & Peach Salad

Prep time: 3 mins | Servings: 3

Ingredients:
- 2 chopped apples
- 1 c. peach
- 1 c. blackberries
- 1 tbsp. lime juice
- 1 tbsp. honey
- ¼ tsp. dried thyme
- ¼ tsp. sugar
- 1 tsp. salt

Directions:
1. Toss all ingredients together and put into serving dish.
2. Serve and enjoy.

Nutritional Information:
Calories: 528 Protein 34g, Carbs 13g, Fat 37g.

Chicken, Apple & Basil Salad

Prep time: 6 mins | Servings: 4

Ingredients:
- 4 c. Basil
- 2 c. chopped Apple
- 2 c. chopped Chicken Breast
- ½ c. sliced Red Onion
- ¼ c. chopped Pecans
- ¾ c. Acai Dressing

Directions:
1. Set 4 salad bowls on the table and add basil to each.
2. Add each of your remaining ingredients as layers on top of the greens.
3. Once satisfied, drizzle each bowl of salad with 3 tablespoons of dressing.

Nutritional Information:
Calories: 269 Protein 34g, Carbs 20g, Fat 8g.

Curried Quinoa Sweet Potato Salad

Prep time: 12 mins | Servings: 6

Ingredients:

- 1 c. Curried Quinoa
- 6 chopped Sweet Potatoes
- 1 c. Water
- ¼ c. chopped Onion
- 1 chopped Celery
- Salt
- Pepper
- 3 boiled Eggs
- 1 tbsp. chopped Dill
- ½ c. Mayonnaise
- 1 tsp. Yellow Mustard
- 1 tsp. Vinegar

Directions:

1. Pour in your potatoes and water into the cooker.
2. Securely close the lid and allow to rise to high pressure over a high flame. Cook for about 3 minutes.
3. Remove the cooker from the flame and cool under cold running water.
4. Proceed to peel and dice potatoes then layer them alternately with celery and onion.
5. Season with salt and pepper then add your dill and chopped eggs.
6. In a separate bowl combine the mustard, mayonnaise, and vinegar then fold the mixture gently into the potatoes.
7. Stir in your cooked quinoa. Chill, serve and enjoy!

Nutritional Information:
Calories: 335.3 Protein 5.5g, Carbs 55.2g, Fat 9g.

Banana Salad

Prep time: 5 mins | Servings: 3

Ingredients:

- 4 sliced bananas
- ¼ c. pineapple sauce
- ¼ sliced onion
- 1 tbsp. lime juice
- ¼ tsp. cinnamon powder
- ¼ tsp. chili flakes

Directions:

1. In a bowl add bananas, pineapple sauce, lemon juice, ad mix.
2. Now season with cinnamon and chili flakes. Serve and enjoy.

Nutritional Information:
Calories: 221 Protein 1.1g, Carbs 57.5g, Fat 0.3g.

Chapter 8 Desserts Recipes

Carrot Cupcakes

Prep time: 15 mins | Servings: 6

Ingredients:

- 1 c. almonds
- 2 c. carrot pulp
- 1 c. chopped dates
- ½ tsp. grated ginger
- 1 tsp. cinnamon powder
- 1 tsp. nutmeg
- ¾ c. raisins

For the frosting:

- 1 c. cashews
- 1 tbsp. water
- 1 tsp. lemon juice
- 6 dates

Directions:

1. In your food processor, mix 1 cup walnuts with 1 cup dates, carrot pulp, 1 teaspoon cinnamon, ginger, a pinch of nutmeg and the raisins, blend and divide this into cupcake cups.
2. Clean your food processor, add 1 cup cashews, 6 dates, a splash of water and the lemon juice and blend these as well.
3. Divide the frosting on the cupcakes, introduce them in the fridge for 1 hour and serve. Enjoy!

Nutritional Information:

Calories: 150 Fat 4g, Carbs 16g, protein 8g.

Dash Diet Doughnuts

Prep time: 10 mins | Servings: 8

Ingredients:
- 3 tbsps. stevia
- 1 c. whole wheat flour
- 1 tsp. baking powder
- 2 tbsps. matcha powder
- ½ tsp. vanilla extract
- ½ c. low-fat buttermilk
- 1 egg
- 1 tbsp. avocado oil
- Cooking spray

Directions:
1. In a bowl, mix flour with matcha powder, stevia and baking powder and whisk.
2. Add buttermilk, vanilla extract, egg and oil and stir using your mixer.
3. Divide into doughnut cavities after you've sprayed with cooking oil, introduce in the oven at 400 degrees F and bake for 10 minutes.
4. Serve them cold.
5. Enjoy!

Nutritional Information:
Calories: 200 Fat 4g, Carbs 26g, protein 12g.

Berries and Orange Sauce

Prep time: 10 mins | Servings: 4

Ingredients:
- 1 c. orange juice
- 1½ tbsps. stevia
- 1½ tbsps. champagne vinegar
- 1 tbsp. olive oil
- 1 lb. strawberries, halved
- 1½ c. blueberries
- 1 chopped peach
- ¼ c. basil leaves

Directions:
1. In a pot, mix orange juice with stevia and vinegar, stir, bring to a boil over medium-high heat, simmer for 15 minutes, add oil, stir, take off heat and leave aside for a couple of minutes.
2. In a bowl, mix blueberries with strawberries and peach wedges, add orange vinaigrettes, toss to coat, sprinkle basil on top and serve! Enjoy!

Nutritional Information:
Calories: 100 Fat 2g, Carbs 20g, protein 4g.

Grapefruit Granita

Prep time: 20 minutes | Servings: 3

Ingredients:

- 1 c. water
- 1 c. coconut sugar
- ½ c. chopped mint
- 64 oz. red grapefruit juice

Directions:

1. Put the water in a pan, bring to a boil over medium heat, add sugar, stir until it dissolves, take off heat, add mint, stir, cover and leave aside for 5 minutes
2. Strain into a container, add grapefruit juice, stir, cover and freeze for 4 hours before serving. Enjoy!

Nutritional Information:

Calories: 80 Fat 0g, Carbs 14g, protein 3g.

Stewed Plums

Prep time: 10 mins | Servings: 4

Ingredients:

- 16 plums
- 1 c. water
- ½ c. coconut sugar
- 5 crushed cardamom pods

Directions:

1. Put water in a pot, add sugar, heat up over medium-low heat, add cardamom, bring to a boil and simmer for 10 minutes.
2. Add plums, stir gently, cover pot and cook for 5 minutes.
3. Leave plums aside to cool down before serving. Enjoy!

Nutritional Information:

Calories: 110 Fat 2g, Carbs 12g, protein 6g.

Lemon Cookies

Prep time: 20 minutes | Servings: 10

Ingredients:

- 1/3 c. cashew butter
- 1½ tbsps. coconut oil
- 2 tbsps. coconut butter
- 5 tbsps. lemon juice
- ½ tsp. grated lemon zest
- 1 tbsp. maple syrup

Directions:

1. In a bowl, mix cashew butter with coconut one, coconut oil, lemon juice, lemon zest and maple syrup and stir until you obtain a creamy mix.
2. Line a tray with parchment paper, scoop 1 tablespoon of lemon cookie mix on the tray, do the same with the remaining dough and freeze for 2 hours before serving. Enjoy!

Nutritional Information:

Calories: 121 Fat 2g, carbs 18g, protein 2g.

Pineapple Bowls

Prep time: 10 mins | Servings: 6

Ingredients:

- 4 c. pineapple pieces
- 2 tbsps. honey
- ½ c. whole wheat and barley cereals
- 12 oz. low-fat vanilla yogurt
- ¼ c. coconut, toasted and shredded

Directions:

1. Divide pineapple pieces into 6 bowls, add yogurt and toss
2. Sprinkle cereals and toasted coconut on top and serve right away. Enjoy!

Nutritional Information:

Calories: 130 ,Fat 6g, Carbs 12g, protein 6g.

Stuffed Peaches

Prep time: 10 mins | Servings: 4

Ingredients:

- ½ c. favorite dried fruits
- ¼ c. toasted almonds
- 4 peaches
- 2 tbsps. graham crackers
- ¼ tsp. allspice
- 2 tbsps. stevia
- ½ c. fat-free yogurt
- 12 oz. canned peach nectar

Directions:

1. Scoop each peach, chop the pulp, put into a bowl, add dried fruits and mix.
2. Also add almonds, crackers, sugar and allspice and stir everything.
3. Stuff each peach with this mix, place them on a baking sheet, drizzle the nectar all over, introduce in the oven at 350 degrees F and bake for 40 minutes.
4. Divide peaches on plates, drizzle pan juices, top with yogurt and serve.
5. Enjoy!

Nutritional Information:

Calories: 130 Fat 2g, Carbs 14g, protein 10g.

Baked Oatmeal

Prep time: 3 mins | Servings: 8

Ingredients:

- 2 c. Quick Quaker Oats
- 1/3 c. Granulated sugar
- ¼ tsp. Salt
- 3 1/3 c. Milk
- 2 medium Eggs
- 2 tsps. Vanilla
- 1/3 c. Brown sugar

Directions:

1. Spray an 8-inch square oven proof glass dish with cooking spray.
2. Heat oven to 350 degrees F.
3. Combine oats, salt and granulated sugar in a large mixing bowl.
4. In another bowl, combine vanilla, eggs and milk and mix.
5. Pour into bowl with oats mixture and mix well. Pour into greased baking dish. Bake into preheated oven for roughly 45 mins or until the center shakes lightly. Remove and place on a cooling rack.
6. Sprinkle dark sugar over the top of the oatmeal.

7. Spread the sugar (using the back of a spoon), into a thin layer across the entire oatmeal surface.
8. Put dish back into the oven and bake until the sugar melts (about 2 – 3 mins). Put oven to broil, and broil for 2 mins, 3 inches from heat until the sugar gets bubbly and slightly brown. (Rotate baking dish to prevent burning).
9. Scoop into bowls and serve.

Nutritional Information:
Calories: 176 Protein 14g, Carbs 35g, Fat 2g.

Whole Wheat Pumpkin Pancakes

Prep time: 15 mins | Servings: 8

Ingredients:

- 2½ c. Pastry flour
- 2 tbsps. Baking powder
- 2 tsps. Ground ginger
- 3 tsps. Cinnamon
- ¼ tsp. Ground cloves
-

- ¼ tsp. Nutmeg
- 2 Eggs
- 2 c. Buttermilk
- 1 c. Pumpkin puree
- ¼ c, Olive oil

Directions:

1. Combine in a large mixing bowl, flour, nutmeg, baking powder, ginger, cinnamon, salt, and cloves.
2. In a second bowl, whisk together, pumpkin puree, eggs, buttermilk and olive oil. Add wet ingredients in second bowl to dry ingredients in the first bowl.
3. Mix until all is incorporated.
4. Grease and heat griddle over medium flame.
5. Use a quarter cup measure to pour batter and let cook until small bubbles form and the sides set.
6. Flip and continue cooking until golden brown.

Nutritional Information:
Calories: 346 Protein 14g, Carbs 34g, Fat 19g.

Tofu Chocolate Cake

Prep time: 10 mins | Servings: 16

Ingredients:

- ¼ c. water
- 300 g block of soft dessert tofu
- One box of super moist chocolate cake mix

Directions:

1. Preheat the oven to 400 degrees Fahrenheit.
2. Using a blender, blend the tofu and the cake mix together.
3. Once these two have been sufficiently blended, add the water and blend again until smooth.
4. Set the mixture into a baking dish. This mixture can also make cupcakes.
5. Cook the mixture to the specifications of chocolate cake mix box.
6. Let the cake cool before serving.

Nutritional Information:
Calories: 190 Carbs 35.8g, Protein 2.9g, fat 4.0.

Low-fat, Sugar-free, Blueberry Cheesecake

Prep time: 15 mins | Servings: 8

Ingredients:

- 2 c. blueberries
- 2c. skim milk
- 2 package sugar-free, fat free cheese cake pudding mix
- 1 container fat free whipped dessert topping
- 1 graham cracker pie shell

Directions:

1. Grab a large bowl and dump both fat free cheesecake pudding mix boxes into the bowl.
2. Take the two cups of skim milk and mix them together till you have a smooth substance.
3. Take half of the mixture and pour it into your graham cracker pie shell.
4. Take half of the blueberries—or whatever fruit you choose—and spread it around the pudding mix. Make sure you press the fruit into it.
5. Pour the rest of the mixture on top of the fruit and spread it out evenly.
6. Take the rest of the blueberries and sprinkle them on top of the pie.

7. Refrigerate the pie for two hours or until it has solidified. You can serve immediately afterward.

Calorie 346.2 fat 7.2g , Carbs 34.9g, protein 5.6g.

Mini Pumpkin Bites

Prep time: 15 mins | Servings: 65

Ingredients:
- 65 reduced fat vanilla wafers
- Dash ground ginger
- Dash ground cloves
- 1/8 tsp. cinnamon
- 2 servings of fat free vanilla pudding
- ½ c. fat free whipped dessert
- ½ c. canned pumpkin

Directions:
1. Take the spices, canned pumpkin, and vanilla pudding and mix it all together thoroughly in a bowl.
2. Take the whipped dessert and fold it into the mixture.
3. Place the mixture into a plastic bag and squeeze it so that it fills the bottom of the bag. Then, clip one of the corners of the bag for easy pouring.
4. Place the wafers onto a cookie tray and squeeze the mixture evenly onto each wafer.
5. Let the wafers chill in the refrigerator for an hour and a half or until they are solid.
6. You can serve immediately.

Nutritional Information:
Calories:17.4 Carbs 3.3g, Protein 2g, fat 7.1g.

Diet Soda Brownies

Prep time: 10 mins | Servings: 12

Ingredients:

- ½ can of your favorite diet soda
- One box of store bought brownie mix

Directions:

1. Preheat oven to 350 degrees Fahrenheit.
2. Instead of using the water, oil, and eggs that is normally used to make brownies, pour the half can of your favorite soda into a mixing bowl.
3. Then, add the box of brownie mix to the bowl.
4. Before placing the mixture into a baking sheet, grease the pan first.
5. Place the mixture into the baking sheet and then cook for twenty minutes.
6. Let cool before serving.

Nutritional Information:
Calories: 114 fat 1.8g , Carbs 138.3g, protein 1.3g.

Chocolate Mousse

Prep time: 5 mins | Servings: 2

Ingredients:

- ¼ c. unsweetened dark chocolate
- 1¾ c. heavy whipping cream
- ½ tsp. orange extract
- ¼ c. cinnamon
- ½ c. whip cream
- ¼ c. dark unsweetened chocolate

Directions:

1. Place all ingredients in a blender.
2. Process until desired consistency is reached.
3. Chill, and top with whip cream and shaved chocolate before serving.

Nutritional Information:
Calories:40 Protein 1g, Carbs 3g, Fat 3g.

Appendix: 21-Day DASH Diet Meal Plan

DAY 1

Breakfast - Very Berry Muesli-24、Easy Shrimp Salad-80

Lunch - Veggie Quesadillas with Cilantro Yogurt Dip-40

Dessert - Carrot Cupcakes-93

Dinner –Buffalo & Ranch Chicken Meatloaf-72

DAY 2

Breakfast - Veggie Quiche Muffins-25、Easy Veggie Soup-81

Lunch - Sweet Roasted Beet & Arugula Tortilla Pizza-41

Dessert - Dash Diet Doughnuts-94

Dinner – Lasagna-60

DAY 3

Breakfast - Turkey Sausage and Mushroom Strata-26、Seafood Salad-81

Lunch - Sunshine Wrap-42

Dessert - Berries and Orange Sauce-94

Dinner - Beef Stew with Fennel and Shallots-61

DAY 4

Breakfast - Bacon bits-27、Caesar Salad-82

Lunch - Southwestern Black Bean Cakes with Guacamole-43

Dessert - Grapefruit Granita-95

Dinner - Grilled Portobello Mushroom Burger-62

DAY 5

Breakfast - Summer Breakfast Quinoa Bowls-28、Greek Chicken Salad -83

Lunch - Southwest Style Rice Bowl-44

Dessert - Stewed Plums-95

Dinner - Chicken Brats-63

DAY 6

Breakfast - Strawberry Breakfast Sandwich-29、Chicken Soup-83

Lunch - Pear, Turkey and Cheese Sandwich-44

Dessert - Lemon Cookies-96

Dinner - Asian Pork Tenderloin-64

DAY 7

Breakfast - Steel Cut Oat Blueberry Pancakes-30、Pumpkin Soup-84

Lunch - Salmon Salad Pita-45

Dessert - Pineapple Bowls-96

Dinner - White Chicken Chili   -65

DAY 8

Breakfast - Spinach, Mushroom, and Feta Cheese Scramble-   31、Spicy Black Bean Soup-85

Lunch - Pesto & Mozzarella Stuffed Portobello Mushroom Caps   -45

Dessert - Stuffed Peaches   -97

Dinner - Brown Stewed Fish-66

DAY 9

Breakfast - Refrigerator Overnight Oatmeal-31、Shrimp Soup-85

Lunch - Fresh Shrimp Spring Rolls-46

Dessert - Baked Oatmeal-97

Dinner - Grilled Cod -67

DAY 10

103

Breakfast - Red Velvet Pancakes with Cream Cheese Topping-32、Mayo-less Tuna Salad-86

Lunch - Washington Apple Turkey Gyro-47

Dessert - Whole Wheat Pumpkin Pancakes -98

Dinner - Baked Salmon-68

DAY 11

Breakfast - Perfect Granola-33、Chestnut Soup-87

Lunch - Pizza in a Pita-48

Dessert - Tofu Chocolate Cake-99

Dinner - Steamed Mussels-69

DAY 12

Breakfast - Peanut Butter & Banana Breakfast Smoothie -34、Pepper Pot Soup-88

Lunch - Heartfelt Tuna Melt-48

Dessert - Low-fat, Sugar-free, Blueberry Cheesecake-99

Dinner - Saucy Chicken-70

DAY 13

Breakfast - Overnight Oatmeal-34、Quinoa & Avocado Salad-88

Lunch - Spinach, Mushroom and Mozzarella Wraps -49

Dessert - Diet Soda Brownies-101

Dinner - Chicken Fried Rice-71

DAY 14

Breakfast - No Bake Breakfast Granola Bars-35、Kale Salad with Mixed Vegetables-89

Lunch - Apple-Swiss Panini-50

Dessert - Mini Pumpkin Bites -100

Dinner - Buffalo & Ranch Chicken Meatloaf-72

DAY 15

Breakfast - Mushroom Shallot Frittata   -36、Cream of Corn Soup-89

Lunch - California Grilled Veggie Sandwich-51

Dessert - Chocolate Mousse-101

Dinner - Shitake & Snow Peas Quinoa   -73

DAY 16

Breakfast - Jack-o-Lantern Pancakes-37、Clam Soup-90

Lunch - Chicken, Apple, and Spinach Salad-52

Dessert - Berries and Orange Sauce-94

Dinner - Chili Chicken Curry-74

DAY 17

Breakfast - Morning Quinoa-37、Apple & Peach Salad-91

Lunch - Coconut Shrimp -53

Dessert - Pineapple Bowls-96

Dinner - Baked Pumpkin Pasta-75

DAY 18

Breakfast - Fruit-n-Grain Breakfast Salad-38、Chicken, Apple & Basil Salad-91

Lunch - Steamed Spinach-54

Dessert - Baked Oatmeal   -97

Dinner - Gruyere and Spinach Casserole-76

DAY 19

Breakfast - Fruit Pizza-39、Curried Quinoa Sweet Potato Salad-92

Lunch - Orange Pineapple Chicken-52

Dessert - Dash Diet Doughnuts-94

Dinner - Roasted Turkey   -77

DAY 20

Breakfast - Flax Banana Yogurt Muffins-40、Banana Salad-92

Lunch - Cinnamon Sweet Potatoes-55

Dessert - Low-fat, Sugar-free, Blueberry Cheesecake-99

Dinner - Honey Garlic Chicken Drumsticks-78

DAY 21

Breakfast - Spinach, Mushroom, and Feta Cheese Scramble-31、Spicy Black Bean Soup-85

Lunch - Chicken Santa Fe-55

Dessert - Whole Wheat Pumpkin Pancakes 98

Dinner - Shrimp Pasta Primavera-79

Made in the USA
Lexington, KY
17 July 2019